T0361633

# CURES OF IRELAND

# Cures of Ireland

## A TREASURY OF IRISH FOLK REMEDIES

## CECILY GILLIGAN

ROWMAN & LITTLEFIELD

*Lanham • Boulder • New York • London*

Rowman & Littlefield
Bloomsbury Publishing Inc, 1385 Broadway, New York, NY 10018, USA
Bloomsbury Publishing Plc, 50 Bedford Square, London, WC1B 3DP, UK
Bloomsbury Publishing Ireland, 29 Earlsfort Terrace, Dublin 2, D02 AY28, Ireland
www.rowman.com

Published by arrangement with *Merrion Press. Tuckmill House, 10 George's Street, Newbridge, Co. Kildare W12 PX39.*

British Library Cataloguing in Publication Information available

**Library of Congress Cataloging-in-Publication Data**

Names: Gilligan, Cecily, author.
Title: Cures of Ireland : a treasury of Irish folk remedies / Cecily Gilligan.
Description: Lanham : Rowman & Littlefield, [2025] | Includes bibliographical
    references and index. | Summary: "Cures of Ireland: A Treasury of Irish
    Folk Remedies is a captivating collection of Ireland's ancient healing
    traditions. It explores a wide range of remedies for ailments from sore
    throats to asthma, and includes the history, rituals, and traditions behind
    these cures, showcasing the secrecy, mystery, and faith involved in Irish
    folk medicine"—Provided by publisher.
Identifiers: LCCN 2024054610 (print) | LCCN 2024054611 (ebook) |
    ISBN 9798881805067 (cloth) | ISBN 9798881805074 (epub)
Subjects: LCSH: Traditional medicine—Ireland. | Folklore—Ireland.
Classification: LCC R498.6 .G55 2025 (print) | LCC R498.6 (ebook) |
    DDC 615.8/809415—dc23/eng/20241202
LC record available at https://lccn.loc.gov/2024054610
LC ebook record available at https://lccn.loc.gov/2024054611

For product safety related questions contact productsafety@bloomsbury.com.

♾™  The paper used in this publication meets the minimum requirements of American National Standard for Information Sciences—Permanence of Paper for Printed Library Materials, ANSI/NISO Z39.48-1992.

For three angels
who believed in this book ~

Andy Rees
Angela Hannigan
Vincent Tucker

Everything on Earth has a purpose,
every disease an herb to cure it,
and every person a mission.

Christine Quintasket
Folklore collector and writer
Native American, c.1885–1936

# Contents

# Prologue

THIS BOOK BEGAN IN 1986 when I was an undergraduate at Cork University. The subject for my final year dissertation was 'Folk Medicine in Ireland ~ Past & Present', and as part of that research I interviewed twenty-eight people with cures. My dictionary defines folk medicine as 'the traditional art of medicine as practised among rustic communities and primitive peoples, consisting typically of the use of herbal remedies ... thought to have healing power'. In rural south Sligo, where I grew up, traditional cures were part of community life; they were well-known and utilised by many. As a child I received a herbal cure for jaundice and my ringworm was healed by the local seventh son. After graduating from college, I continued to have a fascination with the old cures and with Irish folklore generally, but this book lay dormant in my head for almost twenty years.

In 2005 I recommenced my research into folk medicine, initially speaking to the people (or their successors) I had interviewed in 1986. For the following five years I worked to gather as much knowledge as possible on the traditional cures; I strove to gain a comprehensive and analytical understanding of the subject. It took time and perseverance to acquire information regarding cures, as such details are usually passed by word of mouth and are not advertised or publicised. Slowly the names of those with cures began to accumulate, and I started to locate and talk to these people.

In total I interviewed ninety-three women and men, of all ages, with a wide variety of cures, and living primarily in the north-west, where I also reside. These people have cures which are alive and well; some make their cure several times a week, others a few times each year. Those with cures often use the term 'make' the cure to describe the ritual performed and/or the prayers said in the giving of their cure. I spoke to hundreds of people during the years of my research and travelled thousands of miles around Ireland, finding and visiting individuals with cures. Additionally, I documented a selection of holy wells, pilgrimages, clays and stones, all of which are used for healing.

By the opening decade of the twenty-first century huge changes had taken place in Ireland: economically, socially and culturally. These changes included: large-scale movement of people from the countryside to employment in the cities and bigger towns, greater prosperity and educational opportunity for the majority, decline in the power of the Catholic Church, changes to the traditional family structure, decreased fertility rate, increased life expectancy, substantial improvements in healthcare, growing immigration, considerable infrastructural developments, enormous technological advances and greater connectivity to the outside world. Combined, these changes have led to the gradual emergence of Ireland as a modern, educated, affluent, pluralist and multicultural society.

These changes have had an impact on all aspects of Irish life, including traditional cures. Undoubtedly the quantity and diversity of cures has diminished, but interestingly, a significant number of cures continue to exist and to be used. However, the balance between their extinction and survival is delicate. My research (as explored in this book) has found that many of the old cures continue to help and to heal people, and some are thriving.

Innisfree
Sligo

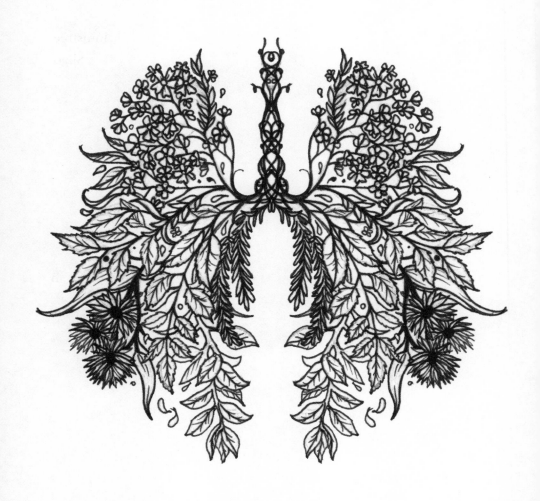

'His sister came and saw that there were 365 different herbs and that each
grew from the part of the body for which it held a cure.'

# CHAPTER 1

# Cures in Ireland Past

🌿

**L**ADY WILDE, POET, FEMINIST, NATIONALIST, folklore collector, and mother of Oscar, wrote in 1888 that the Irish were believed to be the last of the 305 great Celtic nations, and that 'they alone preserve ... the strange and mystic secrets of herbs, through whose potent powers they can cure disease, cause love or hatred, discover the hidden mysteries of life and death'. Some stories from Irish mythology refer to the use of cures, such as in the second Battle of Moytura which took place long ago on a high, windy plain in south Sligo. Lady Gregory, one of the founders of the National (Abbey) Theatre in 1904, learnt Irish and gathered folklore. She recounted how Dian Cécht, the physician and druid of the Tuatha Dé Danann, sang spells over a well nearby and put herbs in it, and the men who had been wounded in this great battle were placed in the water as if dead. 'And not only were they healed, but there was such fire put into them that they would be quicker in the fight than they were before.' Legend says that a large mound of stones, Heapstown Cairn, marks the location of this healing well, which was covered over by the attacking Fomorian tribe.

Nuada, king of the Tuatha Dé Danann, had lost his arm and consequently his title at the first Battle of Moytura (near Clonbur, north Galway) when his army defeated the Fir Bholg people. Metalworker Crédne made him a silver arm. Dr R.M. Blake, delivering a lecture on the ancient Gaelic physicians in 1917, said that it was 'wrought so cunningly that every joint and finger had the mobility of the lost member'. Henceforth, the king became known as Nuada of the Silver Arm. At the second Battle of Moytura his army was victorious, but the king was killed by the giant Balor of the Evil Eye, who came from Tory Island. Local tradition holds that Nuada's grave is the impressive dolmen (portal tomb), known as the Labby Rock, close to the battle site. Marie Heaney tells us that the Morrígan, the battle goddess 'declared victory to the Tuatha De Danann. Then ... she proclaimed peace to the land of Ireland: "Peace in this land From the earth up to the skies ... Honey and mead in abundance And strength to everyone".'

Dian Cécht taught his medical knowledge to his daughter Airmid and his son Miach. However, as the years passed his son's skill outgrew his own. Dian Cécht grew jealous and killed Miach. This was a great loss to Ireland as Miach knew the curative property of every herb. Folklorist Kevin Danaher recalled the end of the story: herbs began to grow on Miach's grave outlining the shape of his body. 'His sister came and saw that there were 365 different herbs and that each grew from the part of the body for which it held a cure.' Airmid collected the herbs and sorted them with care, but her father intervened and scattered them, and ever since Irish folk medicine has been trying to recover this lost knowledge.

A special porridge for the relief of sore throats and colds was believed to have been made by Dian Cécht. This was a mixture of oatmeal boiled with dandelions, hazel buds, chickweed and wood sorrel. Beatrice Maloney documented a 1939 herbal cure from County Cavan which used the same ingredients to treat throat ailments. This indicates that some of the cures might be thousands of years old. Dr John Fleetwood wrote in his *History of Medicine in Ireland* that 'the early Irish physicians were of the priestly or Druidic caste. Their traditions were handed down orally from remote antiquity'.

In the retelling of the *Táin* epic, the two warriors battle on behalf of Connacht and Ulster for the huge and powerful brown bull of the Cooley Peninsula. Thomas Kinsella described this single combat between foster brothers Ferdia and Cúchulainn, which lasted for three days. At the end of each day's fighting the warriors declared a truce, and they shared their provisions and healing herbs. 'Men of healing and medicine came to heal them and make them whole and dropped wholesome, healing plants and herbs into their stabs and cuts and gashes and countless wounds.' Cúchulainn ultimately killed his friend Ferdia on the banks of the river at Ardee in County Louth, a town known in Irish as Áth Fhirdhia, the ford of Ferdia.

There are some references to surgery in Irish mythology. Conchobhar mac Neasa, the king of Ulster, was wounded in the head by a 'brain ball', a missile made using the brain of a fallen enemy. Fínghein, the royal physician, deemed it best to leave the weapon untouched, and Danaher recounted how 'The doctor drew the scalp together over the ball and stitched it with golden thread to match the king's golden hair.' The fourteenth-century *Book of Ballymote* recorded the same doctor and his three apprentices visiting a chieftain whose wound had not healed because of foreign bodies left inside it. Dr Blake stated that by simply listening to the man's groans the young physicians were able to identify the causes: a barb, a reptile and a poisoned dart. The wound was opened, cleaned out, and a cure followed.

Eithne, wife of mac Neasa and sister of Queen Maeve of Connacht, is reputed to have had a successful caesarean section performed on her. Dr Fleetwood recounted the story of Eithne having fallen into a river while heavily pregnant. 'She was rescued in a dying condition. Her side was cut open and a living infant boy delivered.' This incident is understood to have taken place at Tenelick in south Longford and the river still bears her name, though in an anglicised form, the Inny.

Ireland was ruled by native tribes or clans (families) whose power and territory ebbed and flowed over the centuries. These regional chieftains governed using the Brehon laws, which Fleetwood described as having been 'first promulgated several hundred years before the birth of Christ. Their growth was gradual ... kings and judges ... added their own contributions ... They were abolished in the reign of James I ... but many of them were respected even by the Anglo-Irish up to the middle of the seventeenth century.' Under Brehon law physicians were awarded special status, some form of medical registration existed, and they were paid (often in cows) 'according to the social grade of the wounded person'.

Ireland was never invaded by the Romans, which was probably significant for the survival of traditional cures and healing practices. Celtic scholar Jeffrey Gantz wrote that, 'By virtue of its westerly and isolated geographic position, this island remained free of Roman colonization; thus, Irish society did not change appreciably until the advent of Christianity.'

## Healing Monks and Hereditary Physicians

Christianity came to Ireland in the fifth century, and slowly began to impact on the beliefs and behaviour of the people. The first holy men brought with them the written word and during the following centuries monastic scribes painstakingly created ornate, beautiful manuscripts. They wrote down the ancient, oral tales of Ireland, but most likely retold these stories in a way that reflected their own patriarchal, Christian perspective. Kevin Danaher noted that monasteries became the focal point for the teaching and practice of medicine; care of the sick and the poor was organised within them. Many monks became expert in the production and usage of herbal cures, ointments and drinks.

Niall Mac Coitir, in his book *Irish Wild Plants*, has written that 'In ancient Ireland ... herb and vegetable cultivation was particularly associated with monasteries ... All the produce of these gardens was grown to promote well being: medicinal herbs and nourishing vegetables.' The sites of old monastic settlements are still considered by some to be important locations for the gathering of wild, healing plants. A man in north Leitrim whom I interviewed in 1986 and whose family had a famous herbal cure for shingles, told me that 'they used to say there was a cure for every disease in the monastery field [nearby]'.

Trepanning, or trephining, was the surgical removal of pieces of bone from the skull to relieve pressure on the brain, and it appears to have been carried out in Ireland in previous centuries. John Fleetwood wrote that major surgery like this would have taken place in the monasteries. He referred to St Bricín of Cavan carrying out this operation in AD 637 on a man wounded in battle, by removing 'the injured portion of the skull and brain ... and on his recovery his intellect and memory were more powerful than ever'. In 1969 author and film-maker Bob Quinn witnessed an elderly farmer perform this procedure on Clare Island (west Mayo). He recalled, 'I saw an islander conducting brain surgery on a sheep! The operation, called "trepanning", is an ancient and well-attested procedure for relieving painful pressure on the brain ... colloquially, "the head-staggers".'

The early Christian period was a relatively peaceful time in Ireland, but all this changed dramatically with the arrival of the Vikings at the close of the eighth century. The wealthy monasteries were repeatedly attacked and plundered by the merciless Norsemen, who had sailed and rowed from Scandinavia in their sleek longboats. Two hundred and fifty years later the descendants of these fearsome warriors had settled in Ireland, and founded coastal trading towns like Dublin, Wexford,

Waterford, Cork and Limerick. Academic Nora Chadwick alluded to the Battle of Clontarf (1014) in her study *The Celts*: 'This great battle put an end to the Viking supremacy in Ireland ... the Celtic way of life survived, and so ensured the continuation of the basic farming economy.'

The Anglo-Normans came to Ireland in the twelfth century and for the following four hundred years they tried to colonise the country. The east, in particular the area known as The Pale (around Dublin and north to Dundalk), became their stronghold. But the noble Gaelic families continued to rule much of Ireland, holding onto their lands and wealth, and supporting their clans' poets, musicians, storytellers and physicians. Dr Fleetwood has written that 'From about the tenth century until the foundation of a formal medical profession, medicine in Ireland was practised by hereditary physicians whose families were attached to specified nobles and chieftains. Younger members learned from their elders and were expected to carry on the family tradition.'

Mac Coitir stated that 'all the Gaelic septs (or clans) had hereditary medical families linked to them', and that the O'Lee, O'Shiel, O'Hickey, O'Meara and O'Cassidy families were among those closely associated with the art of healing. Often these hereditary physicians possessed a family book of medical knowledge. Dr Patrick Logan believed that many of the cures which have survived have their origin in these medieval textbooks, and in later eighteenth- and nineteenth-century medical manuscripts. Patrick Logan made an immense contribution to the study of traditional healing practice in Ireland, much of which is contained in his classic book *Irish Country Cures* (first published in 1972). Born and bred in south Leitrim, he worked as a doctor in Dublin, and over a forty-year period he collected and investigated cures. Most of them were told to him by his patients and work colleagues, who came from every part of Ireland.

The late Dr Patrick Heraughty, of The Mall, Sligo, also had a great understanding and appreciation of Irish folk medicine. He speculated that if one generation of the hereditary physician family was less capable, an element of superstition or magic would have been introduced to cover up their shortcomings. This reasoning may help to explain the use of Cassidy's Rag to cure sick animals in Ulster, often believed to be under the influence of the evil eye. In the early 1900s Henry Morris recorded farmers getting a piece of coat lining from anyone with the surname Cassidy and burning this fabric under the animal's nose to ensure a cure. Three centuries earlier the O'Cassidys had been the hereditary physicians to the Maguires of Fermanagh. They had lost their status when the noble family was dispossessed of their lands. However, a link between the family name and a healing capability remained.

Geoffrey Dent's 1968 article in *Ulster Folklife* reported that 'Throughout the north of England there is still some evidence of the tradition that anything originating in Ireland had the power of healing.' He found that an ability to heal had been regarded as inherent in the Irish and that methods of medical treatment were more likely to be successful if applied by a native of Ireland.

Ireland, like most of Europe, was struck by the Black Death in the middle of the fourteenth century. This was a pneumonic and bubonic pandemic spread by fleas and rats. It arrived in the port towns and quickly moved inland. The death toll was highest in the urban centres where the Anglo-Irish population was concentrated. The *Local Ireland Almanac 2000* review of the millennium lists it as a significant event, and states 'that up to half of the population of Ireland may have been wiped out before 1400'.

The Irish monasteries, which had been centres for care and medicine, were dissolved in the sixteenth century by King Henry VIII. The Gaelic chieftains struggled to hold onto their power until the early 1600s, at which point England gained almost complete control of Ireland and continued to rule the country for the next three hundred years. The penal laws (1691–1829) took away the power and wealth of the native population in a number of ways, including by not allowing Catholics (the majority of Irish people) to buy or inherit land, to be educated abroad, or to vote. Historian J.C. Beckett stated that the essential purpose of these laws 'was not to destroy Roman Catholicism, but to make sure that its adherents were kept in a position of social, economic, and political inferiority'.

# CHAPTER 2

# Cures in the Nineteenth and Twentieth Centuries

※

I N THE EARLY 1800S THE traditional cures were the only form of medicine available to most of the population, who were poor, landless peasants. People had to rely on themselves, their families and communities for the maintenance of their health. Dr Logan wrote extensively on Irish folk medicine and he believed that the traditional cures 'were probably as effective as the official remedies before the twentieth century and certainly they were cheaper and more readily available'. The people worked on the land and were healed by the land. Over the centuries a comprehensive knowledge of the medicinal value of herbs had been accumulated, to the benefit of humans and animals. David Allen and Gabrielle Hatfield documented the ethnobotany of Britain and Ireland, and they have written that 'the main mass of people depended for everyday first aid ... [on] local plant remedies ... a herbal repertory built up over the generations by trial and error ... their knowledge transmitted by word of mouth'.

Much of the nineteenth century was a dark, traumatic time for

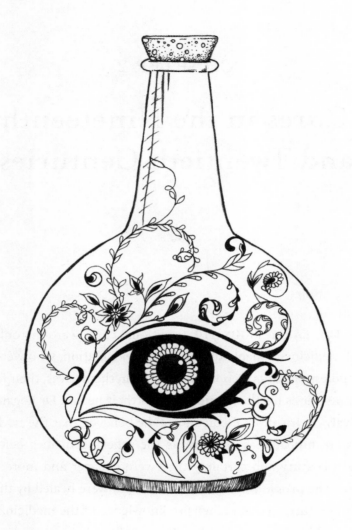

*Biddy Early, the famous wise woman from east Clare, was remembered as independent, generous and good-looking. She could see the future in the bottle given to her by the fairies.*

the people of Ireland. A typhus epidemic in 1817 lasted for two years, affecting all parts of the country, and an estimated 65,000 people died. In 1832 an outbreak of cholera claimed up to 50,000 lives; it spread quickly from county to county, killing swiftly and indiscriminately, unstoppable in the slums of Dublin. My local town, Sligo, was a busy port at the time and it was particularly badly affected, with up to 10 per cent of the population (1,500 people) dying in less than one month. Charlotte Thornley, Bram Stoker's mother, lived in Sligo and survived the epidemic. It is thought that the stories she told her young son of this nightmarish time, and of people being buried alive, partly inspired his famous novel *Dracula*. Interestingly, Danaher found that garlic (a deterrent to vampires!) had been used to prevent the spread of cholera 'by hanging its cloves in a little bag around the neck or binding them under the armpit'.

On 6 January 1839 Ireland was hit by a hurricane, known in folk memory as the Night of the Big Wind. Although loss of life was relatively small, the ferocious and unexpected tempest devastated the countryside, destroying crops, livestock and the hovels that many lived in. Six years later when the people were recovering from this natural disaster, the man-made catastrophe, the Famine began. After five years of widespread famine the population had decreased dramatically, due to death on a huge scale and emigration. Hundreds of thousands of refugees boarded coffin ships to North America, fleeing hunger and disease, desperate to survive and searching for a better life.

Frank Mitchell and Michael Ryan recall, in their book *Reading the Irish Landscape*, that 'During the famine years (1845–51), about eight hundred thousand people died and twice as many emigrated. The heart was knocked out of Ireland and the population continued to fall from a maximum of eight million without interruption until 1930, when it was only four million and Ireland was one of the emptiest countries in Europe.' The population of our country has never recovered from this momentous human tragedy; official figures for 2022 show that the population of the island of Ireland (the Republic and Northern Ireland) was just over seven million.

Much of the knowledge and expertise of traditional healing must have been lost with these people. Allen and Hatfield believed that the mass emigration to the USA and Canada had a profoundly negative effect on folk medicine; they wrote that, 'For the Irish, the physical severance from country ways that resulted was so abrupt and wholesale that their traditional herbal lore must inevitably have been largely forgotten.'

The Famine had a devastating impact on the Irish language also, as the areas that were most affected by it and had the biggest death toll, were where the language was strongest. In *Mapping the Great Irish Famine*, we are told that the 'highest concentration of Gaelic speakers was in the west of Ireland, economically the least developed parts of the country. The Famine killed many Irish speakers and compelled many others to emigrate ... [It] reaped a grim harvest of men, women and children.' E. Estyn Evans, writing in his reference book *Irish Folk Ways* (1957), likewise believed that the Famine had led to major changes in the rural economy and landscape; it was, he said 'a great social watershed and it marked the end of an era that might well be termed prehistoric'.

## Wise Women

Mac Coitir recalled that in the nineteenth century, 'The "Herb Woman" or Bean na Luibheanna was a well-known member of every Irish community, and her knowledge of the medicinal properties of plants made her someone both respected and feared.' Lady Wilde (pen name Speranza) called these women fairy doctors, and described them as curing 'chiefly by charms and incantations, transmitted by tradition through many generations; and by herbs, of which they have a surprising knowledge'. Her husband Sir William Wilde, a distinguished doctor, antiquarian and Irish speaker from Castlerea, County Roscommon, collected folklore too and her published work is most likely a result of their combined research.

Dr Logan wrote of the fairy doctors, that 'there can be no doubt that many of them were brilliant psychologists ... had the essential quality of a successful healer; they understood that the patients were worried and needed to be reassured ... sincerely believed that they had power to heal and to help ... [and were] wise enough to know that nature is a great healer'. From her research in Ireland, folklorist Nancy Schmitz of Québec found that healing powers were more likely to be attributed to people who were viewed as marginal in the community; they were often women who were elderly, widowed and independent, or Travellers (nomadic people). These women were known as the *bean feasa* (knowledge/wise woman) or the *bean leighis* (medicine woman). Schmitz described the wise woman as 'a person whose access to "power" is greater than that of others in society. Her function is to remedy damage or illness untouchable by the usual medical remedies, and to act as an intermediary between the ordinary world and the "supernatural", similar to certain shamans.'

The best-known wise woman in Ireland at this time was Biddy Early, who was born in the tumultuous year of 1798 (the Irish, supported by France, rebelled unsuccessfully against English rule). She lived near Feakle in east Clare. Biddy had a great knowledge of wild plants and their healing properties, probably handed down to her from her mother. She was believed to have spent time with the fairies, and consequently she was able to diagnose and cure illnesses caused by them. She had a special bottle, given to her by the fairies, which helped her to heal and in which she could see the future. Biddy was extremely popular with the public and was visited by thousands of people, including Daniel O'Connell, over many decades. Her reputation as a powerful healer grew and grew, and was known the length and breadth of Ireland. Biddy Early was consistently bullied by the clergy, denounced from the pulpit and excommunicated from the Catholic Church. However, she grew prosperous, was married four times and lived a long life. She was remembered as a good-looking woman, strong-minded, kind and generous.

In 1902, over twenty years after Biddy's death, Lady (Isabella Augusta) Gregory set out from her home (Coole Park), with her pony and trap, to visit Mrs Early's cottage. She had heard many stories about this famous healer from her tenants in south Galway. 'When I got back at nightfall to the lodge in the woods I found many of the neighbours gathered there, wanting ... to know for certain if she was dead. I think as time goes on her fame will grow and some of the myths that always hang in the air will gather round her.'

When I was a child in the 1970s, her name was often mentioned in my home. I remember we still had a lot of respect for and some fear of this celebrated wise woman, who had died one hundred years previously. She was buried at Feakle in an unmarked grave. I visited Biddy Early's ruined cottage in 2005, and I found little offerings of jewellery and flowers on a windowsill there. The house and garden on a low hill have long been abandoned to nature. The small, reedy lake below is supposedly where a priest cast the magic bottle following her death, and despite various attempts, to date it has not been recovered.

Fortunately, women in Ireland who were healers and midwives did not suffer the same horrific fate as women healers in many other parts of Europe. Mary Condren writes of the genocide that was enacted against women, and particularly wise women, accused of witchcraft by misogynistic, patriarchal Christian churches and states. The number of women who were brutally murdered is unknown, but it could be as high as nine million over four hundred years, from the 1300s to the 1700s. To quote Condren, 'The story of the witches, or the genocide of women healers, is one of those epochs in human history so devastating and beyond comprehension that it has scarcely been touched by historians.' Some men were also accused of witchcraft, tortured and killed.

Ann Oakley explored the history of childbirth, and the demise in power and status of the traditional midwife or wise woman. She believed that 'The existence of the woman-midwife-witch-healer challenged all three of these hierarchies ... church over laity, man over woman, landlord over peasant ... [therefore she was seen as] a threat to the established social order.' Jeanne Achterberg examined the historical role of these women in her book *Woman as Healer*, stating 'since women were not officially allowed to study medicine, it was widely accepted that their information could only have come from the devil ... "she is a witch and must die" ... The machinery of Church and state had conspired to create "the shocking nightmare, the foulest crime and deepest shame of Western civilization ...".' Today, in the twenty-first century, we still unquestioningly read *fairy* tales to children that often include a terrifying, evil woman, a *witch* character. These stories are, of course, not reflective of real life.

In modern Irish *cailleach* is generally taken to mean a witch, a derogatory name. But it can also be translated as nun (the veiled one), wise woman or fortune teller. Gearóid Ó Crualaoich, in his *Book of the Cailleach*, looked at the traditional stories associated with the *Cailleach Bhéarra* from the Cork/Kerry region. He describes her as:

> an archetypal figure of Irish myth and legend ... the hag/mother-goddess of Beara ... omnipresent guardian of her territory ... the epitome of longevity ... [an] association between her and the forces of wild nature ... the spirit of the high ground, of mountain and moor ... [a] fertile power that is as vast and as untameable as the wild, wide landscape.

Ó Crualaoich draws a link between the pre-Christian *cailleach* (goddess) and the women of more recent centuries who helped and healed their communities: 'the services of the *bean ghlúine* (midwife), the *bean feasa* (wise-woman) and the *bean chaointe* (keening-woman), to name three human female personae whose *cailleach*-inspired (and derived) performance of service to the community was so essential.'

The *cailleach* was also the name traditionally given to the last sheaf ceremoniously cut at the end of the harvest, which was brought home, preserved and sometimes plaited. In certain areas grain taken from this special sheaf was the first to be sown the following spring. Anne O'Dowd, a former curator of the National Museum of Country Life in Mayo, recalled that 'Once it was taken to the home, the last sheaf ... became an object imbued with a certain mysticism ... it was believed to be good for the health and wellbeing of cattle, the productivity of hens, the luck of the household and the welfare and safety of people.'

## Fairies and Changelings

The fairies or *na sióga* are believed to be the Tuatha Dé Danann, a mythical, magical race who ruled Ireland long ago and were followers of the fertility goddess Danu (also known as Áine). Following their defeat by the Milesians they went to live underground inside the fairy forts and beneath the sea in splendid palaces. Tara expert Michael Slavin wrote that 'The final confrontation between the Dé Danann and the Milesians was on the Plain of Teltown, north of Tara [the royal seat]. There the Dé Danann were overcome ... they agreed that while the newcomers should rule on the earth, they would rule in the Otherworld.' The fairies are also known as *na daoine maithe* (the good people) or *na daoine uaisle* (the noble people); they are immortal, and they love music, song and dance.

They are most active and closest to humans during the great festivals of *Bealtaine* (May Day, the first day of summer) and *Samhain* (Hallowe'en, the first day of winter). Nora Chadwick explained that '*Samhain* (1 November) was the beginning of the Celtic year, at which time any barriers between man and the supernatural were lowered.' The other two very important days in the year's cycle, which have their origin in pre-Christian Ireland, are *Imbolg* (great belly), the first day of February and spring (fertility), and *Lughnasa*, the first day of August and autumn (harvest).

The feast of *Bealtaine* was marked by the druids. They lit a huge fire on the Hill of Uisneach in County Westmeath, which was believed to be the centre of Ireland. On the eve of May Day, yellow May flowers (marsh marigolds) were placed on the doorsteps and windowsills of homes and byres to protect the inhabitants from the fairies for the coming year. This practice continues in pockets of the north-west, and some people stick a branch of gorse out of an upstairs window of their house to welcome summer. Niall Mac Coitir, in his book on the folklore of Irish trees, has written that on May Day the golden-yellow gorse blossoms were 'brought into the house, or placed over the door or in the thatch, for luck and to "bring in the summer" ... a symbol of wealth and the fertility of the land ... linked with the goddess of the land'.

Midsummer was another extremely significant celebration in pagan times. The High King lit the first fire on the Hill of Tara, and once this was done other fires and festivities commenced across the land. Many Irish people still light a fire to celebrate midsummer (21 June). The Catholic Church Christianised this ancient festival, moved it to 23 June, and renamed it St John's Eve or, as it is more commonly known, Bonfire Night. Folklorist Bríd Mahon recalled that 'Herbs gathered at this time of year were said to be especially powerful. St John's Wort (hypericum) ... was known as the fairy herb because of its curative properties ... It was used for the treatment of rheumatism and bruises, and a remedy for the "airy fit" (an attack of depression).'

Douglas Hyde, from north Roscommon, became the first President of Ireland in 1938. He was an academic, a linguist and a renowned collector of folklore. He contributed to anthropologist Walter Evans Wentz's book on Celtic fairy-faith, writing that 'The *Sidhe* or Tuatha De Danann were a people like ourselves who inhabited the hills ... and who lived there a life of their own, marrying ... banqueting or making war ... A belief in them formerly dominated the whole of Irish life.' Edmund Lenihan, a gatherer of folklore and stories, noted in 1987 that 'A mere generation ago every field and gap, even bushes, had a name ... Dotted among their fields were forts, blessed wells, fairy hills, each with its own story passed down through the generations, a living proof that we share this ground with others [the fairies] who are best left alone.'

This belief is strong in rural Ireland and as a result many national monuments, especially megalithic tombs, have remained intact. Unfortunately, fairy (ring) forts have fared less well. These are the remains of our ancestor's homes, circular areas, enclosed by earthen banks and ditches, and often located on hills. The *Atlas of the Irish Rural Landscape* states that over 45,000 ringforts have survived. However, many more have been destroyed by farm modernisation, urban expansion and road construction. The place names remind us of their presence, *ráth*, *lios* and *dún*. Also, *caiseal* or cashel, which were settlements surrounded by strong stone walls. To cut down a fairy tree (often a lone hawthorn) or to damage a fairy fort is still guaranteed to bring misfortune upon the offender and their family. This can take the form of financial ruin, a terrible accident, physical or mental illness, and even death.

In 1911 Evans Wentz recorded the testimony of a Mayo priest, who told him that:

near Ballinrobe there is an old fort which is still the preserve of the fairies ... the farmers wouldn't cut down a tree or bush growing on the hill ... some time ago in laying out a new road the engineers determined to run it through the fort, but the people rose almost in rebellion, and the course had to be changed.

There is a little hawthorn tree on the edge of the highway at Latoon in south Clare, close to the five-star Drumoland Castle hotel. When a new road was being constructed there in 1999, a local *seanchaí* (storyteller) warned the County Council that if this fairy tree was removed, bad luck would follow. So, following no doubt much deliberation, the carriageway was diverted sideways and the fairies were left in peace!

The cry of the banshee (*bean sí*, woman fairy) was much feared as it foretold the death of a family member. Peter Kavanagh (brother of Patrick, the poet) collected folklore and in 1958 he wrote that she was 'A fairy woman who warns certain Irish families of an impending death by wailing for three nights before the house of the person who is about to die'. The banshee was reported as being a small old woman or young and beautiful, both were embodiments of the *cailleach.* Patrick Logan understood that she was particularly known to lament the passing of those from noble families and he believed she was possibly a personification of a war goddess from much earlier times.

Belief in the changeling was prevalent in nineteenth-century Ireland. It was used as an explanation for the high levels of infant and maternal mortality, and poor health. These deaths and illnesses were more likely caused by poverty, malnutrition, untreated childhood diseases, tuberculosis and postnatal depression. It was thought that fairy women were unable to have healthy babies or to suckle them.

Therefore, the fairies abducted babies and children, and women who would care for them, as well as young women to be fairy brides; they left behind a weak, sick, *fairy* version of the human. Occasionally the fairies took men also, especially if they were musicians. W.B. Yeats presented a romantic picture of the changeling in his poem 'The Stolen Child' written in 1886:

> Come away, O human child! To the waters and the wild
> With a faery, hand in hand,
> For the world's more full of weeping than you can understand.

One of the most infamous cases concerning this belief in fairy abduction of humans was that of Bridget Cleary in 1895, midst the fertile farmland of south Tipperary. Bridget was twenty-six when she suddenly became unwell, probably with pneumonia, but her family believed her to be a changeling and a local fairy doctor was consulted. She was forced to drink herbs in milk, shouted at, beaten, doused in urine, and finally set on fire by her husband. It was felt that these actions would drive the fairy out of her body. As a result of this abuse Bridget died and she was secretly buried in a shallow grave.

Her husband and extended family were tried for the crime, and he was convicted of manslaughter; he served fifteen years and subsequently disappeared to Canada. Over one hundred years after Bridget's death, Angela Bourke told this young woman's tragic tale:

> The story of Bridget Cleary is firstly one of 'domestic' violence ... Their society was strongly patriarchal ... After seven years of marriage, the Clearys had no children ... and a childless marriage was unusual, even shameful. The fairy-belief tradition ... It is precisely a way of labelling people as

not quite human, and serves to rationalize the ambivalence or hostility felt towards those who are different.

Bridget Cleary was laid to rest nearby at the village of Cloneen, in an unmarked grave.

In the west of Ireland, the practice of dressing small boys as girls continued into the twentieth century. It was a ploy to fool the fairies who were believed to be more likely to take away male children. Bob Quinn noted that in the past in northern Holland 'The Friesians also dressed young boys in skirts to ward off the fairies, who were apparently not interested in girls, a tradition exactly duplicated in the Aran Islands [Galway Bay].' In his exploration of the wealth of folklore from the Great Blasket Island off west Kerry (abandoned in 1953), Pádraig Ó Héalaí found that fire was used as a protection against the fairies: 'it was said ... that if a woman jumped over the flames of the bonfire on St John's Eve, her children could never be harmed by the fairies'.

I came across a Scottish reference to the changeling in a folk tale from the Orkney Islands. Tom Muir recalled that 'The wise woman said that her bairn [child] had been taken by the fairies and they had left one of their own in its place as a changeling.' Logan tells us that the changeling is also a character found in Icelandic folk stories. Ireland, Scotland and Iceland have been linked by the sea for centuries and this has surely led to an intermingling of our folklores.

Richard Breen researched the concept of the *piseog* (a charm or spell), which was the practice of actively trying to inflict bad luck on somebody. A *piseog* was laid in secret, and often by hiding something perishable (like eggs or meat) near your enemy's house or on their land. Breen explained that 'The logic of the belief is that as the piseog decays so will the good luck of the farmer.' Similarly, if an animal died the carcass could be thrown into a neighbour's field thereby transferring the bad luck to them.

Some people were thought to possess the evil eye, generally those at the fringes of society, such as women with children out of wedlock and those born illegitimate or not baptised. Richard Jenkins stated that there was a clear link 'between the evil eye and deviance from the community's moral code'. Those with this affliction were believed to be able to cause bad luck or sickness to humans and animals just by looking at them, or by not using the customary greeting 'God bless you'; hello in the Irish language is *Dia dhuit*, which translates as God to you. Lady Gregory was told by a woman from the Aran Islands in 1898, about 'The time my son got the pain, he came in roaring ... Father Mc Evilly told me ... He said a woman that was carrying [pregnant], and that was not married ... she might put the evil eye on you.'

In a 2001 article in the folklore journal *Béaloideas* Professor Michael Doherty of the School of Veterinary Medicine, University College Dublin, documented the contemporary belief held by a small number of Irish farmers in the negative effect of the evil eye or blinking on their animals. He wrote that 'some people in Ireland today believe that individuals – particularly strangers coming onto a farm for the first time – have the ability to "blink" an animal, resulting in the appearance of disease or a drop in milk production'.

## Cures in the Twentieth Century

By the end of the 1800s modern medicine had started to develop in Ireland, with a corresponding decline in folk medicine. Jenkins has written that at this time, 'Hospital, doctors and veterinary surgeons replaced the wise-men and -women, while a new, and equally mysterious set of causal categories, "germs", "infection", etc ... replaced the witches and fairies.' The Irish Universities Act of 1908 consolidated the existing third-level colleges and created an overarching National University of Ireland. These universities had medical faculties; in the early 1900s women accounted for just 1 per cent of their students; one hundred years later in 2014, 57 per cent of medical graduates in the Republic of Ireland were women.

In 1903 philanthropist Lady Rachel Dudley collected money to start a district nursing service along the western seaboard, in some of the poorest regions of Ireland, particularly Connemara. An article in the *Women's Studies Review* (1997) described the work of these nurses as having been 'extremely hard and demanding, especially the midwifery ... her only transport was a bicycle over rough unpaved roads, and on foot across bogs and mountain: she had to go out in all weathers day and night ... being on call seven days a week'. The Lady Dudley nurses continued to provide care for the sick of west Galway until they were absorbed into the emerging public health system in 1974.

From the late 1800s and throughout the twentieth century, people gradually moved from the countryside to the growing towns and cities in search of work, opportunity and prosperity. The power and influence of the Catholic Church steadily increased, education levels rose, and a financially comfortable middle class emerged. Ireland became a Free State in 1922 following the War of Independence with Britain. Northern Ireland, which had been created a year earlier, remained part of the United Kingdom. Ireland became a Republic in 1949.

In the 1960s the country started to modernise slowly and our entry into the European Economic Community (EEC) in 1973, the forerunner of the European Union (EU), was to be hugely significant and beneficial to the people, especially to farming families. The population of the nation began to grow from the late 1960s, as did the economy, and there was a gradual increase in the standard of living for the majority. As a result of these changes a way of life in rural Ireland, which had altered little for hundreds of years (particularly in the poorer west), was coming to an end.

For most of the twentieth century many Irish people, especially those in the countryside, had limited access to modern medicine and continued to utilise traditional cures for themselves and their animals. This was how some of the people I interviewed described this dependence. A farmer with the cure of the burn said, 'if you go back thirty years ago there was no running to a doctor … people really depended on cures'. A grandmother in south Sligo had a burn cure too and she told me, 'we used to have a cure for everything … doctors and vets were never needed, and cures were common knowledge'. There was a woman in County Cavan with a herbal cure for whitlow (a finger infection). She felt that in the past people rarely went to a doctor or a hospital: 'country areas always had cures … they made up their own concoctions and cured themselves'. She also said it is reckoned that 'everything that grows, there's a cure in it'.

A fisherman in Donegal made a prayer cure for bleeding. He believed his cure to be very old, that it went 'back probably to famine times … that's when I think most of these things were made up to help people … they had nothing else, they had no money, they had to do something'. I spoke to a Roscommon woman in her late seventies with a popular cure for migraine. She had been making her cure for more than forty years and inherited it from her mother, who was given it 'by an old lady that was seven years old at the time of the Famine … she lived in a mud house in the bog … about a mile [away]'.

An elderly man who had a cure for jaundice said that not so long ago, 'a lot of people had more faith in cures'. They did not like or could not pay for a doctor to come to their house. I interviewed a man with cures for colic, burns and vertigo, and he told me that years ago 'cures existed in every townland … there was somebody … who could cure everything … the doctor was for when you were dying'. He thought that as income levels increased and people could afford to go to doctors, the cures decreased: 'poverty kept the cures … riches killed them'.

Anne MacFarlane has looked at the changing role and status of women as health workers in Ireland. Her findings were supported by interviews with older people (average age seventy) in 1995–96. The interviewees believed that the use of traditional medicine had declined significantly over their lifetimes, in tandem with the rise of modern medicine. One person summed up this change by saying 'there came a time when there was a doctor and more modern times. It was like going from the horse to the tractor. It was a lot easier to go to the chemist than go out to the field and pick and mix.'

Anthony Buckley, curator of the Ulster Folk and Transport Museum, carried out considerable research into the folk medicine of Northern Ireland and in 1980 he published an article called 'Unofficial Healing in Ulster'. At that time, he believed the traditional cures were strong in his area and he stated that 'Despite the considerable successes of modern scientific medicine in the last hundred years, there seems to have been only a slight abatement in the popularity of unofficial remedies in Ulster.'

Allen and Hatfield wrote in 2004 of 'the greater scale on which reliance on folk medicinal herbs has persisted in that country [Ireland] till very recently ... the substantial degree of autonomy that Irish folk medicine seems to have enjoyed'. They believe that 'Ireland's lengthier history of poverty and, especially in the west, greater remoteness from the Classical herbal tradition ... have compelled in this respect a self-sufficiency that has been both more extensive and longer-lasting.'

## A Land Rich in Folklore

In Ireland we are very lucky to have one of the best folklore collections in Europe. This is primarily due to the work of the Irish Folklore Commission, established in 1935 by the fledgling state to record and preserve the folklore of the nation. It was driven by Séamus Ó Duilearga (Delargy), who was joined by Seán Ó Súilleabháin, and a small team of dedicated and hard-working folklorists. Intrepid collectors were sent forth on bicycles, armed with cumbersome recording devices, to conduct fieldwork in the remotest parts of Ireland. During the 1940s Séamus Ennis, the famous uilleann piper from Finglas (Dublin), gathered music, song and lore in the west, in both the Irish and English languages.

In addition, questionnaires on a wide range of subjects (customs, beliefs and recollections) were distributed to people within communities across the country; these were volunteers who had an interest in the oral tradition. The archive of the Commission (1935–71) was to evolve into the National Folklore Collection, which is now housed in University College Dublin and in 2017 became part of UNESCO's Memory of the World Register.

One of the jewels of the collection is the folklore gathered by the school children of Ireland over a two-year period, 1937–39. A total of 50,000 children in 5,000 schools across the Republic, with the support of their teachers, amassed 740,000 beautifully handwritten pages documenting local history, traditional belief and practice. The enthusiastic scholars interviewed their families and neighbours, especially the old people, for stories of fairies and ghosts, crafts and customs, herbs and remedies, and lots more. Folk medicine was a subject area which got a great response; thousands of cures, for animal and human ailments, were recorded. This wealth of material, which is known as 'The Schools' Collection', has been conserved and catalogued, and can now be accessed online.

# CHAPTER 3

# Cures in Ireland Today

I INTERVIEWED NINETY-THREE PEOPLE WITH cures between 2005 and 2010. I began with the twenty-eight people I had interviewed in 1986 or whoever they had given their cure to. Roughly one third were still making their cure, another one third had passed on their cure, and the final one third had died and taken their cure with them. I then went looking for others with cures; I wanted to investigate as many types as possible and to get a comprehensive picture of traditional healing in Ireland at the start of the twenty-first century.

This was a slow process. Often, I got into my car and went searching; sometimes phone calls proved helpful to track down a cure. I gradually acquired the names of many people with possible cures, usually with vague directions as to where they lived. Every time I interviewed someone, I asked them did they know of others who had cures. Family, friends, neighbours and work colleagues who were aware of my interest also passed on names to me. I compiled a list of over three hundred people with cures and it is still growing.

My interviews took the form of a qualitative study, a series of questions which I felt were the most important and relevant to the

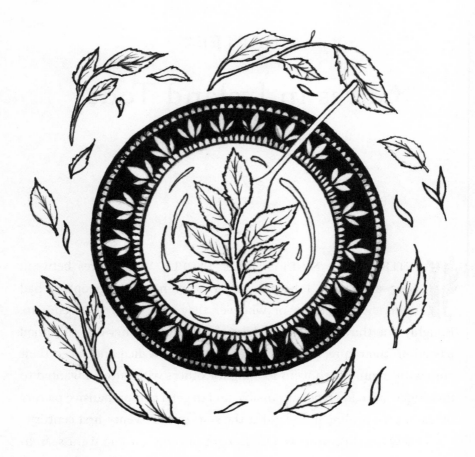

*Cures I came across in my research, included: covering a wound with a cobweb to stop bleeding, nettle soup in the springtime for blood pressure, eating young dandelion leaves for gallstones and drinking honey in warm milk at bedtime for a good night's sleep.*

subject. The answers supplied in these interviews have formed the core of this book. I stopped interviewing when I felt I had a broad understanding and record of the cures that exist in contemporary Ireland, and when much repetition of information was occurring. Other traditional cures for people and animals probably (and hopefully) exist in Ireland today, but I did not come across them. My research was extensive and thorough; I left no stone unturned!

Most of the people I approached were willing to speak to me, to share their experiences and thoughts on their cure. However, many of them did not want to draw attention to themselves or their cure; they preferred to keep their identities private. I have respected people's wishes and not used their names, and have generalised where they live.

The cure tradition is surviving in Ireland, as documented in this book, and it remains relatively strong in the north-west (particularly in rural areas) where I conducted most of my research. Sr Nora Smyth of Armagh investigated and collected cures from people (especially the elderly) over a twenty-year period, and in 2002 she published an eclectic little book, *Going For The Cure*, based on her research in the north-east. She found that in her region the folk cures were 'still part and parcel of everyday life ... alive and well'.

## Who Makes Cures?

An analysis of those I interviewed shows that all sorts of people make cures: women, men, and children, old, middle-aged, and young, rural and urban dwellers, Catholics, Protestants and those with no religion. They are ordinary people, with this additional aspect to their lives. Those with cures are unprofessional and unqualified; they have no formal medical training. Most people have one cure, some a few. They make their cures independently and in isolation. There is no obvious link between people with traditional cures. To shed greater light on this analysis, I have looked more closely at a few factors: location, age, gender and economic influences.

Location is a significant factor as cures are more common in rural Ireland; I heard of very few city people with cures. Over 60 per cent of my interviewees lived in the countryside and many of them were farming (part- or full-time). The cures have their roots in the land, and this is where they have survived and thrived for generations. More than 20 per cent of those I interviewed lived in villages and small towns. Interestingly, about 14 per cent were from big towns and thereby classed as urban folk.

Cures are often associated with elderly people. This is because people usually hold onto their cure as long as they can and will only pass it on to the next generation when they are in poor health or too old to keep making it. Rather than viewing the cure as dying because it is in the hands of an older person, it can be interpreted that the cure is surviving and that it is ready to be passed on to a younger person, to get a new injection of life and energy. Almost 10 per cent of my interviewees were in their eighties, the biggest cohort was the fifty to seventy age group (45 per cent), and just 5 per cent were in their twenties. It seems that the Irish cure tradition respects and values age, maturity and wisdom.

The cures I documented were divided equally between women and men. But in general, I found that more men than women have cures, based on the names I gathered. My research showed a difference of about 12 per cent. Why does this disparity exist? I am unsure of the answer. A common stipulation when cures are passed on is that the gender must change each time (woman to man, to woman), therefore the sexes are equally represented. In the past women were more closely associated with healing in Ireland, as highlighted by the *bean feasa* (wise woman) tradition. I do not think a patriarchal bias exists in traditional Irish healing practice today. Smyth discovered in her fieldwork that it was primarily women who had cures and she wrote, 'It is not surprising that the majority of the curers are women. Traditionally, the woman is the person most concerned with the health of the family.'

Social class, income level or employment status do not appear to influence the making of cures. People with cures are rich, financially comfortable and poor, and they have every type of work; they are farmers, builders, politicians, artists, electricians, bus drivers and shopkeepers. The global financial recession took place during the period of my interviews, and it contributed to an abrupt and dramatic end to Ireland's economic boom. This undermining of the country's economy led to major social, community and family upheaval. Irish unemployment was just over 4 per cent in 2005 and by 2010, when I finished my research, it had jumped to almost 14 per cent. The unemployment figure for 1986, when I conducted my initial study of the cures, was close to 17 per cent, also a very bleak time for Ireland. I conclude that the traditional cures are generally independent of economic influences; people will make their cure irrespective of their employment status or financial circumstances.

## What are Cures For?

The group of people I interviewed had 119 cures collectively for thirty-nine (human and animal) ailments; these included asthma, headaches, sprain, ringworm, thrush, shingles and colic. Irish traditional cures tend to be for minor or chronic conditions, though I encountered cures for skin cancer and the heart too. Heart disease has long been a serious health concern in Irish society. According to government statistics for 2018, almost 30 per cent of deaths were due to diseases of the circulatory system. Dr Patrick Logan had similar findings in his exploration of the old cures. He noted in 1972 that 'Folk medicine provides treatment for all the ordinary and obvious diseases, but it does not deal with certain parts of medicine'; for example, he believed that, 'Treatments for internal cancers are very rare.'

My research found that there are basically two types of cure being used in Ireland currently, faith and herbal. Faith cures are by far the more common; they were almost 80 per cent of those in my study. Fewer herbal cures exist; they accounted for just 20 per cent of the ones I documented. Faith cures centre around prayer, whereas herbal cures utilise healing plants, but often a prayer or a blessing is incorporated. Beatrice Maloney, recording cures in Cavan in the 1970s, discovered that people thought it very important to partner the plant with the prayer; ''tis little good the herb will do if you don't know the verse', she was told.

Examples of the two types of cure are as follows. I interviewed a woman in her sixties who made a faith cure for toothache; she was a writer, mother and homemaker. She lived in a small town in County Sligo, but was given this cure by her father-in-law from rural north Leitrim. The cure was a short, secret prayer, just four lines. Most people telephoned her and she said the prayer for them immediately. They did not have to be physically present and she did not need to know their name. She had had this cure for over thirty years and helped 'hundreds of people'. She needed to pass it on to a man, most likely her son. When I asked her what was the source of the cure, she replied, 'I think it's faith ... the same God that cured the lepers is still here ... that's what cures the people.'

I also spoke to an elderly woman with a herbal cure for gout, which she had been making for twenty-five years. She explained the process: 'I have to gather the herbs when they're in season and dry them ... and store them then for the winter.' She used two herbs that she collected locally (their identities are not revealed): 'I like to get them as clean as I can ... I would go to quiet lanes.' When a cure was requested, she simmered the herbs in water, allowed the liquid to cool overnight, then squeezed the plants with her hands and strained the mixture twice. She put the herbal liquid into a one-litre plastic bottle. The people who received her cure were told to keep it in the fridge and to 'take a small, half glass before their breakfast [fasting] every morning ... until it's gone'. There were no prayers accompanying this cure. 'It's totally herbal ... I'd have ... faith in the herbs,' she said.

I regularly came across variations of the same cure. In the Irish healing tradition, each cure is unique and particular to the individual making it; even if two cures appear to be very similar, there are almost always small differences, as demonstrated by the cure for burns. Two people I met with this cure lick the burn, but one also blessed himself and asked the injured person to bless themselves three times.

The cure of the sprain is another example of the use of slightly different approaches to achieve the same goal. A retired woman in the midlands had this cure. She rubbed the sprain and said a prayer. The cure was made over three days, which could either be Monday, Thursday and Monday, or any three days in a row. Depending on which option was taken the prayer would also vary. A Tyrone farmer with a similar cure would start by asking the person to bless themselves. Then, he touched their sprain, making the sign of the cross on it three times and said a blessing silently each time. It was a quick procedure which could take place anywhere, in his house or the farmyard (for animals). He too repeated the ritual for three days.

People with cures usually have a strong adherence to all the elements of their cure. They tend to accept unquestioningly the rituals involved, and to make it as it was given to them or as the tradition dictates. Minor changes are made to cures, small personal variations, but essentially the cures remain unaltered; therefore, they have survived for decades, even centuries, almost intact.

## Why Use Cures?

Why do people get cures? I did not ask those who avail of cures this question. However, following my interviews with those who make cures, I believe there are a number of answers to this question. Most notably, the cures have played an important role in Irish society in the past, and a continuity of respect for and interest in them survives. Also, many people who get cures have faith in them; they believe they will work. In addition, cures exist within communities and farther afield, and if someone needs a cure and they are aware of its location, or if one is recommended to them, they might find it simpler, easier and cheaper to take this route rather than go to a general practitioner (GP), pharmacist or vet.

Having said this, most people in Ireland today rely primarily on modern medicine to address their health concerns. They may look for a cure for a minor problem, but if the condition is more serious, they will usually visit a doctor or hospital. Sometimes, people take a cure in tandem with medical treatment. Others get cures as a last resort; they have tried modern medicine without success and they have nothing to lose. The reality is that those who use cures combine the two approaches to healing, the traditional and the modern, to suit their needs. Nora Smyth reached a similar conclusion following her research in Northern Ireland, writing that 'it has not been unknown for conventional medicine and folk medicine happily to co-exist side by side'.

I always asked my interviewees why people got their cure and didn't go to a doctor. The following are a selection of the responses I received. One woman with a cure for shingles said that many people have been to the doctor before coming to her, and been prescribed with 'cream to rub on … and tablets, which are very expensive'. Another woman who had a few cures for animals, including pink eye and sprain, told me that some people try the cure before the vet because they believe in the cure and it is cheaper. A man with a back pain cure thought that he was the second choice for most people. They have already been to a doctor, but their pain continues; 'some have gone to the doctors and they've failed

... or they mightn't want taking tablets'. Similarly, a person who made a cure for hiatus hernia felt that people generally try the doctor before his cure: 'they tend to go to the doctor ... get their operations ... then come for the cure, when everything doesn't work'.

## Cures I Have Gathered on My Journey

These are cures I came upon during my research. I do not know their medicinal values and I am not recommending them. I am documenting them as part of the folkloric tradition of Ireland. The same applies to all the cures and information contained in this book.

Arthritis: dandelion tea made from the leaves in spring and sweetened with honey, or simmer wild garlic leaves in milk, strain and drink, or eat parsley, or apples, or take a seaweed bath.

Asthma: drink goat's milk, or *carraigín* (seaweed) boiled in water.

Back pain: make a poultice with nettle leaves and apply, or press the back into an oak tree.

Baldness: rub the head with a raw onion, or relax with seaweed on the head!

Bedwetting: give the child a teaspoon of honey at bedtime.

Bleeding: to stop the flow, cover with a cobweb.

Blood pressure: nettle soup in springtime (nettles indicate fertile soil), or young wild garlic leaves as a salad, or stop, rest and enjoy nature.

Boils: apply honey, or a white bread poultice (yeast batch bread soaked in warm milk, place on the boil).

Bowel problems: eat wild bilberries, raw or cooked.

Bruise: place raw meat on it.

Burn: cover with buttermilk, or honey or houseleek (split open the leaf), or fresh cow dung, or torn cabbage leaves.

Burn, inside mouth: hold cream in the mouth.

Car sickness: pick mint, bruise it, and keep it in the car.

Chest problems: drink goat's milk, or honey in hot water, or blackcurrant tea, or eat spring dandelion and wild garlic leaves, or tie a strip of red flannel (woollen) cloth around the chest and keep it there until the condition improves.

Chilblains: soak the feet for fifteen minutes in your own urine, dry them, but do not wash off the urine, or rub on fasting spit, or cod liver oil, or onion juice.

Cholesterol: spring nettle tea.

Cold: drink buttermilk, or blackberry and elderberry syrup diluted with water, or eat cooked turnip, or honey.

Cold sore: rub a gold wedding ring around it, or rub with a dock leaf.

Complexion: apply a face pack of oatmeal and buttermilk, or for beautiful skin, wash your face in the May Day morning dew, at sunrise.

Corn/bunion: walk barefoot in the bog, or bandage a fatty rasher to it, or wrap in unwashed sheep wool, or rub with ivy leaves, or houseleek, or dandelion milk (sap from the stem).

Cough: make rosehip syrup (rich in vitamin C), dilute with hot water and drink.

Detox, springtime: young nettle soup, or wild garlic as a soup or eat the leaves as a salad.

Earache: simmer half an onion in water for one hour, then place the warm onion in a sock and apply to the ear.

Eczema: drink goat's milk, or apply a mixture of buttermilk and honey, or a bran poultice.

Gallstones: dandelion tea or eat the young leaves as salad.

Gout: eat parsley, or nettle soup, or apply honey.

Hair growth: wash with nettle tea.

Hangover: eat some honey and drink lots of water.

Headache: to be free from headaches for a year, get a haircut on Good Friday.

Hives: rub with dock leaves.

Infection: use a white bread poultice to draw it out.

Infertility: visit a *sheela-na-gig* (also known as a *cailleach*, the goddess), which is a stone carving of a female figure displaying her vulva, often sited on the walls of old churches or castles; there are about one hundred still to be found around Ireland.

Insomnia: honey in warm milk at bedtime, or dandelion leaf tea.

Kidney stones: eat parsley, young dandelion leaves and blackcurrants.

Liver tonic: spring dandelion leaves as a salad.

Measles: young nettles as a tea, or briefly simmer the leaves in water, strain and eat.

Midges: rub elder leaves or bog-myrtle on the skin to deter them, and avoid sweet food.

Mumps: simmer young nettles in milk, strain, add honey and drink, or pass the child three times under a donkey that has never been ridden.

Nettle stings: rub the affected area with ribwort, or with a dock leaf, whilst saying three times, 'Dockin, dockin, cure me nettle!'

Ringworm: make the sign of the cross on the infection with a gold wedding ring (do this for three days), or bless the ringworm with straw from the Christmas crib, or apply cider vinegar.

Ringworm, on cattle: cover with cow dung, or seaweed or wild garlic.

Scalds: apply egg white, or grated raw potato and a layer of honey.

Shingles: steal water (used to cool down the iron) from a blacksmith's forge, but make sure nobody sees it being stolen; this water must be rubbed on the shingles for nine mornings.

Sore throat: boil *carraigín* in water, sweeten the liquid with honey and drink, or boiled *duileasc* (seaweed) in milk, or rosehip syrup in hot water with honey, or just honey.

Spots: apply your own spit.

Sprain: crush some comfrey leaves and bandage them around the damaged limb, or apply a chickweed poultice.

Stings, bees/wasps: apply onion juice, or houseleek, or dandelion milk, or a bread soda/water paste, or cider vinegar.

Stye in the eye: using a blessed, gold wedding ring, make the sign of the cross over the stye for nine days, or look through a wedding ring with the affected eye and bless yourself three times, or bathe the eye with cold black tea.

Sunburn: apply buttermilk.

Thorn/splinter, to draw it out: bandage a white bread poultice to the skin.

Tired feet: put alder leaves in your shoes, or walk barefoot on the beach.

Tonic: mix three teaspoons of cider vinegar and three teaspoons of honey in a glass of water, and sip slowly.

Tooth/gum infection: use warm, salty water as a mouthwash.

Ulcer: eat blackberries and honey, or apply torn cabbage or dock leaves.

Verruca: apply dandelion milk, or cider vinegar.

Warts: if you come upon a rock with water collecting in it, rub this water on the wart three times, or apply sand found under seaweed, or raw potato, or pierced sloe berries, or rub dandelion milk or onion juice on the wart, once a day for nine days.

Whooping cough: pass the child three times under a white horse, or completely around (under the belly and over the back) of a female donkey three times.

Wounds: apply crushed plantain, houseleek or yarrow leaves.

Wellbeing: climb a hill, walk in the woods, or swim in the sea, you will feel healthier and happier!

# CHAPTER 4

## FAITH CURES

# Hearts, Strokes, Heads, Sprains and Healers

OST OF THE TRADITIONAL CURES that are to be found in contemporary Ireland can be regarded as faith cures. They partially or totally consist of prayers and their success is generally attributed to God. Many Irish people still hold strong religious beliefs; religion was an integral part of their upbringing (in particular their education) and it has been a core institution of Irish society for decades. In the 2016 census just under 80 per cent of the population identified themselves as Catholic; this figure was higher in rural areas and lower in the cities. However, the number of Catholics in Ireland is steadily declining; it had decreased 6 per cent since the census five years previously and there was a corresponding increase in those who said they had no religion, almost 10 per cent in 2016.

Despite this trend Ireland is still a Catholic country; Mass

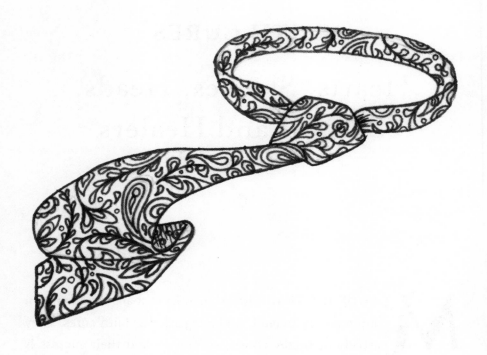

*A middle-aged woman used her late father's tie to make the head fever (migraine) cure.*

attendances are dropping, but church funerals, weddings and baptisms remain the norm. At times of difficulty and crisis in people's lives, such as when they are sick, people turn or return to their religion for support. I believe that the saying of prayers, by those receiving and giving cures, can often provide reassurance and hope, and can enhance the healing process. Focus on the physical ailment may be lessened, and the psychological and spiritual aspects of the individual may be activated to contribute towards their cure.

## Hearts

There was a cattle farmer in his sixties who lived in north Tyrone, close to the border with Donegal. He had well-known cures for heart fever and sprain. This man had a broad understanding of what heart fever was. He told me that it was more than a physical heart problem. It had a psychological dimension which included stress, anxiety and depression; he described it as 'a big, heavy weight on the heart'. He said heart fever was more prevalent in the autumn and spring, 'the fall of the leaf and the bud'.

People telephoned to request the cure and while he was talking to them, he would start the ritual. He had a measuring tape laid along a kitchen worktop; he placed his elbow at the start of the tape and put his forearm down flat along it. He saw the position the tip of his middle finger reached, and he lifted and placed his elbow at this point. He lay his forearm along the tape a second time and again took note of where his middle finger extended to. He placed his elbow at this point and repeated the action for a third time. Following these three forearm lengths, the final position on the tape was noted and here a little cross was left.

To make the cure he repeated the procedure, but this time as he was doing it, he said the person's name as part of a blessing. He said three blessings to correspond with the three forearm lengths. The result of this second measurement indicated whether the person had heart fever. If the three forearm lengths had not reached the cross, he believed the person did not have the problem. But if his fingertip was touching or had gone beyond the cross, 'that tells me ... there's something not right with them'. If this was the case, he asked the person to phone him in three weeks and he would again make the cure for them, 'and not before the three weeks is up'. He said that the second time he made the cure the heart fever would hopefully be gone. If not, he would repeat it a third time, seven days later.

An important part of this man's cure was talking and listening to people. 'I'd talk to them then, to find out what was ... bothering them ... they'd open up to you.' Some people were lonely, many depressed, and they told him of financial worries and marital breakdown. If the cure was for a young person, he preferred to speak to them rather than their parent. This aspect of the cure took time, 'sometimes twenty minutes', but he gave generously of his time. Occasionally, he advised people to go to their doctor, 'because I would know there's something underlying'.

His was an extremely popular cure administered to 'hundreds' of people every year. He got calls every day; they telephoned him from all over Ireland and even from South Africa. He would not take money for his cure: 'no ... you don't take anything for God's work,' he said. However, his late wife, who gave him the cure, used to pass any money she was given for the cure to the local hospice, so he would do likewise. He told me that the cure helped him cope with the loss of his wife and that it had had a very good effect on his life: 'it gives you a good feeling whenever you can ... help people along the path of life'. He believed that his cures 'come from the healing Jesus ... I'm just an instrument ... doing God's work.'

I interviewed a retired man living in rural east Sligo. He had two cures, for heart fever and head fever (headaches). Both cures involved quite complicated rituals and it usually took ten minutes to make them. For the heart fever one, he would ask the person coming for the cure to bring pinhead oatmeal with them. Then he filled a small glass to the top with the oatmeal, levelled it off with a knife, and covered the glass with a white handkerchief. He turned the glass upside down and moved it anti-clockwise around the person, pressing it to their clothed body at five different locations: at the centre of the chest, under the left armpit, at the centre of the back (heart height), under the right armpit, and returning to the centre of the chest. As he moved around the body, he slowly said a blessing and the five parts of the blessing coincided with the five parts of the body he was touching. This procedure was repeated three times.

Then, as he continued to hold the upturned glass of oatmeal to their chest, he prayed aloud. He said fifteen prayers, five Our Fathers, five Hail Marys and five Glory Bes. As he was praying, he thought about the saint of the cure and Josephine, the woman who gave the cures to him. He said there were three people involved in his cure apart from himself: the saint, Josephine and the person getting the cure. Once the prayers were completed, he removed the cloth from the glass. If there was a problem with the person's heart some of the oatmeal would have disappeared and there was usually an indent in the oatmeal at the side of the glass.

One of the most fascinating elements of this cure was that the person receiving it played an active role. They had to take home the oatmeal that remained in the glass, and cook and eat it as soon as possible. He told me, 'They're not allowed to let anyone pass between … the bag of oatmeal and themselves.' To achieve this he suggested they keep the oatmeal close to their body, maybe in their pocket. He made his cure on Mondays and Thursdays, and each time the person returned he repeated the ritual. They kept coming to him until the oatmeal in the glass remained unchanged and there was no indentation in it. This was taken as a sign that the heart problem had healed. He felt that God caused the healing to take place in his cures: 'It's all belief, belief and faith … belief in God.'

Fifteen kilometres away there was a man who made a similar cure. He acquired it from his late mother and the cure had been in his family for at least five generations; it dated from the mid-1800s. He also said prayers as he was making the cure, but he kept them secret and they were in Latin; Catholic Masses were said in Latin until 1965. Patrick Logan documented a comparable cure for the heart in Leitrim in the 1960s, except in that case an eggcup of oatmeal was bandaged to the sick person's chest and they were sent to bed, as 'it must remain undisturbed for the nine days'.

## Blood Pressure and Strokes

I spoke to a middle-aged man who lived among the rolling hills of east Fermanagh, not far from the border with Monaghan and the Republic. He had a cure for blood pressure (high and low) and heart fever: 'It's the same cure for all three problems,' he clarified. 'I think a lot of people probably would be attending a doctor … maybe they've tried tablets and it hasn't worked … then they'll come to me for the cure.' It was a prayer cure, but he did not want to tell me exactly how he made it; this element of secrecy was 'part of the cure'.

Anyone who wanted his cure just needed to ask for it. He liked people to write to him and explain their problem; he would then make the cure especially for them. He told me that as he was making the cure he had to concentrate: 'I would be making the cure, probably nearly every evening … I [would] be on my own … quietly,' and that it could take up to an hour to complete. 'I write back to them and let them know that I've the cure made.' He made the cure once, unless he was asked to repeat it. He accepted money for his cure, but he told me, 'I make the cure for them regardless of whether they give me money or not.' It varied from person to person; some gave money, some did not, and some preferred to donate to charity.

There was a man (mid-forties) who farmed cattle and sheep on the fertile land of north Kildare. He had a famous family cure, a bottle, which helped many problems, most notably strokes. He said that the majority of people wanted the cure for 'strokes, blood pressure and circulation'. He told me of a woman who had been on life support following a stroke. She was given his cure and recovered; 'that's a regular occurrence'. His bottle had also been used to help arthritis, sciatica, headaches, Bell's palsy, vertigo, eczema and depression.

This was a very popular cure and large numbers of people came for it every week, from every region of the country. The day I interviewed him he said, 'If you were here ... half an hour ago ... there was about forty people ... Sunday ... there could be one hundred or two hundred people.' Cars queued along the little road leading to his farm. People tended to phone in advance to get information about the cure, usually from his wife.

The preparation of the cure was a secret; however, he did tell me that, 'There is herbs I pick up around the farm, holy water and prayers ... I make up a big bottle.' He freshly prepared a large bottle the days he made the cure, which were Sunday, Monday and Thursday (between noon and 1 p.m.). He administered the cure to people in a bedroom in his house. Initially, they discussed what the problem was; if it was for the individual present, he would make the cure for them. If the cure was for someone elsewhere, he gave them a small bottle of the cure to take away, with instructions for applying it.

He always made the cure in the same way irrespective of the problem. To start the ritual he blessed himself, then dipped his finger in the cure bottle and rubbed the water on the person at a number of places on their body: the forehead, both sides of the face, back of the neck, wrists and ankles. He rubbed each body part three times, and before each rub he dipped his finger in the cure water; it was necessary to touch their skin. If the person had had a stroke and 'their speech is affected, I rub it on their voice box,' he added. To finish the ritual, he said three Hail Marys and blessed himself, 'In the name of the Father, the Son, and the Holy Spirit, Amen.'

This was a pleasant, practical man, who focused on getting the job done, yet giving everyone individual attention. People returned twice more to see him, on the specified days, to have the procedure repeated and the cure completed. The three visits could be spread over three weeks, which was helpful to those travelling long distances. If people felt they needed a second cure they could return after three months.

He gave a little bottle of the cure water to those who wanted to bring it to someone in hospital. He directed them to apply it using the same procedure as he would, and to come back for the second and third bottles. There were also three conditions which had to be adhered to. The cure could only be applied by a man. It was to be rubbed on the sick person the same day as it was collected, before midnight. And most interestingly, once the cure was made, the water remaining in the bottle had to be taken outside and disposed of in a place where nothing (human or animal) would cross over it: 'pour whatever is left ... into a hedge, a tree ... down a wall ... where nothing walks'. He emptied whatever water remained in his large bottle in a similar way when all the cures for that day had been made. I believe that this aspect of the ritual was to ensure that the illness was transferred to the earth; this concept is important in the Irish cure tradition.

Seventeen years earlier he had inherited the cure, along with the family farm, from his father. The cure could only be passed along the male line of the family, which is probably the reason why he stipulated that a man must administer the cure to someone elsewhere. He felt it was important that the cure stayed within his family and that if it 'went outside that circle, it wouldn't work'. He was a young man, but when the time comes, he will most likely pass it to a nephew.

I was told that the cure took up a lot of his time: 'I'm farming here as well, it's very time-consuming ... [we] don't get many holidays!' He was a very generous man. He accepted no money personally for his cure and if people left him some, 'I give it to charity.' I asked him what did he believe was the source of the healing in his cure. His reply was that it was a faith cure, but also that it was made 'with good intentions ... from the heart'.

I came across the Padre Pio glove in 2005, while visiting a relative in a large hospital in the north-west. It was being used to help a stroke patient, and was rubbed on the man's head and hands by his daughter as a prayer was said. Padre Pio was an Italian priest (1887–1968) who became an esteemed Catholic saint because he allegedly had the stigmata (the same wounds that Jesus had on the cross) on his hands, feet and side. This old, brown, woollen glove had been worn by Padre Pio over his bleeding and bandaged hand; it is now a relic believed to have curative powers. The glove was protected behind plastic in a leather wallet, accompanied by a prayer to the saint and a brief explanation of its history. It is in the possession of a family from the north-east and they lend it to those in need of healing.

## Headaches

I interviewed an elderly woman in rural north Roscommon, the mother of eleven children. She had a cure for head fever: 'In the olden days it was called head fever, now they call it migraine,' she explained. It was a pressure in the head, at the back of the neck, over the temples; 'everyone differs ... some do have a very bad pain,' she said. Generally, she made the cure in the entrance hall of her cottage; people sat on a chair there, and the procedure took 'about five minutes'. She talked to

people and reassured them before she began; 'I do tell them to relax …
[they have] a lot of stress in their lives.'

To begin the cure she would bless herself, then ask the person to
say one Our Father and three Hail Marys, and she would say one Our
Father, five Hail Marys and one Glory Be. Next, she laid her hands on
their head for a short time; 'I would feel if it was swollen.' Then, using
a long, black ribbon she took two measurements of the person's head,
from the back around to the forehead and from under the chin to the
top of the head. She made two knots on the ribbon to indicate these
measurements. If the two knots were in a similar place, she knew that
the person was well, but if the knots were a distance apart, they had
head fever.

People came to her three times to finish the cure, on Mondays and
Thursdays, and during daylight hours. She requested them to say one
Our Father and three Hail Marys every day for the duration of the cure,
and for two weeks afterwards. At the end of the first visit, she would tie
the black ribbon around the person's head. She instructed them to wear
it continuously until the three visits had taken place. She said people
could take it off temporarily if they were having a shower, combing
their hair or going to Mass. By the third visit, when the measurements
were repeated, the two knots on the ribbon should be touching and this
meant that the cure had been successful. She warned people, 'They're
not to measure … their heads themselves … they break the cure.' She
would then remove and keep the ribbon, wash it and use it for another
person.

Her cure, which she had been making for over four decades, was
well-known. The number of people looking for it varied from week to
week: 'It depends … you might have five one day … no one for a month
… I had three yesterday.' She helped young and old, 'a lot of children',
many of them strangers. 'They come miles', from Kildare, Dublin and
as far south as Cork. She thought most people had been with a doctor

before they tried her cure. Occasionally, someone came with a tumour and she said, 'I would tell them they'd have to go back to the doctor.' This woman had great faith in her cure and in God: 'I believe that God helps me to help them.'

I spoke to a friendly woman in her sixties who lived in the centre of a large town in the north-west. She made a cure for head fever too, but she did not believe this condition to be a headache; rather she told me, 'it's more of a heaviness ... a very, very heavy head ... and a hot feeling'. She had had this cure for twenty-five years; it originally belonged to her late father and she used one of his ties to make the cure: 'I do it with my father's tie ... Daddy told me how to do it and I still keep to that.'

To make the cure, the person would sit and she generally stood beside them. She blessed herself, then laid the tie on top of their head and said three blessings. Using the tie, she took two measurements of the head, in the same way as the north Roscommon woman. She said a blessing three times as she took each measurement. Holding the tie, she then leant her hands firmly on the person's head, 'in three different positions, forehead, middle and back'. She told me that following this ritual, which had to be repeated three times, 'you can know if the head is open' and if so, the person has head fever. 'As you do the cure ... the next day, you can know by the tie ... if it's closing in.' She would then ask the person to say a prayer, 'whatever little prayer they like, every night for nine nights'. When they had left, she would say nine prayers for them, three Hail Marys, three Glory Bes and three Our Fathers.

To complete the cure, people visited her three times, on Thursdays and Mondays only, and 'you're supposed to do it before the sun sets'. But if some were unable to come to her for three days, she repeated the procedure three times when she first met them. She believed the source of the healing was God, and she also felt that the cure, 'it's coming from me ... it's coming from my father ... it's coming from the Gallagher man [who originally had it]'. She said, 'I never refuse anybody ... I always find time to do it.' Some people were in a hurry, but more sat down for a chat, and 'I always ask ... would they like a cup of tea?' She did not take money for her cure; 'it's nothing out of my pocket to do the cure ... just say a prayer ... or light a candle for me'.

There was a man in east Sligo who made a headache cure in a similar way to these two women; he had cures for heart fever and strain too. He was a straight-talking, middle-aged farmer and builder, and was very clear that someone who wanted the cure must ask personally for it: 'The person themselves has to ask for it ... it's no good if another person asks me.' The cures were given to him by his mother and he lived in her former home, which helped ensure continuity and the survival of the cures. He needed to pass them on to a woman, and he told me that 'with God's help' he would choose wisely, so that the cures would be 'kept alive'. He had great faith in his cures, but he felt that those receiving them did not necessarily have to believe in them: 'It doesn't seem to matter ... maybe someone belonging to them has some faith in it?' he speculated. When I asked him why he made his cures, he replied, 'If you're able to do any little bit of good for anyone, aren't you as well doing it.'

Dr Logan wrote of the headache cure, that 'the ritual of measuring and squeezing and the repetition will probably be of great benefit to the patient. Carried out by a healer who understood people and sympathised with them, this treatment would surely be as helpful as the best modern psychotherapy.' One hundred years before I documented these cures for the head and heart in east Sligo, Lady Gregory had recorded equivalent ones from the Gort area of south Galway. A Mrs Quaid had informed her, 'I have a charm myself for the headache ... I used to put on a ribbon from the back of the head over the mouth, and another from the top of the head under the chin and then to press my hand on it, and I'd give them great relief and I'd say the charm.' And a Mrs Creevy recounted, 'I saw her fill the bowl with oatenmeal, and she

HEARTS, STROKES, HEADS, SPRAINS AND HEALERS

tied a cloth over it, and put it on the heart. And when she took it off, all the meal was gone out of one side of the bowl, and she made a cake out of what was left on the other side, and ate it. And the boy got well.'

## Sprains and Strains

In south Cavan there was a middle-aged woman farming and working as a dairy quality controller. She had the cure of the strain. 'It's for anything muscular ... ligaments, tendons ... any part of the body.' She told me that she made the cure for anyone who requested it, 'but I don't guarantee it will work ... I ask them are they sure it's a strain ... I tell them I'm not a medical person.' Her cure combined prayer and touch: 'You just say the prayer and ... concentrate on the area where they say they have the pain ... you use your hands to stretch the affected area.' She touched their skin or through their clothing, 'it will work either way'. She said two prayers (which she kept secret) as she was touching the person. Some people felt heat from her hands; 'I don't [experience heat], but they do ... they often say ... how warm your hands are ... they can feel heat in the area.'

Her cure was quick: 'five minutes', and she could make it any time; usually, she saw people at her home in the evening after finishing work: 'They'll ring you in advance ... you know how many you have to come.' The cure had to be made over three consecutive Mondays and Thursdays, and she believed this aspect of the ritual was very important: 'You have to do it three in a row, if you miss a day ... if you break it, you have to start again.' Normally three visits sufficed, but if people felt they needed a second cure, they were welcome to return.

I interviewed an elderly, Leitrim woman who had cures for jaundice and strain. She was well-known for her strain cure which she made for people and animals, cattle, horses and donkeys. People could either come in person to receive the cure or they could telephone her and she would make it for them. If the cure was for an animal, she asked the name of the owner, what type of animal it was, and where the injury was located.

When someone came to her house, she started by making the sign of the cross with her hand over the strained part of the body while saying a blessing; she repeated this ritual three times. Next, she prayed as she continually touched the strain: 'I'd rub it … all the time while I was making the cure.' She said three common prayers, the Creed, the Our Father and the Hail Mary, and a special prayer for the cure of the strain. This procedure was repeated on two other days to finish the cure.

She had been making the cure for thirteen years and her late husband gave it to her; it was in his family for at least three generations. She believed she could give the cure to more than one person: 'You can pass it on to anyone that wants it.' At some point in the future, she intended to give it to her son; at the time, she was content to keep making the cure; 'I'll keep doing it, while I'm fit.'

I also spoke to a woman in her thirties, living in rural west Sligo, with a sprain cure; she was the manager of a shoe shop in a local town. She told me that she made her cure for any area of the body that was sprained, mostly wrists and ankles, 'a few backs'. She was unable to help broken bones and advised people to go to a doctor if she thought it was more than a sprain. The person with the injury generally sat and she knelt beside them; 'you kneel down, you bless yourself'. Then she rubbed the sprain three times and made the sign of the cross four times over it with her thumb. As she was touching the person she silently prayed, common prayers and her own prayers; 'I talk to God,' she said. To end the ritual, she blessed herself. The person getting the cure had no prayers to say.

'You repeat that process three times and then that's the cure finished.' People had a choice as to how to do this. She could make the cure over three days and repeat the short ritual each day. But the more popular option was for her to repeat the ritual three times in one visit; 'most people ... they travel such a distance ... you can make it three times there and then ... and it suffices'. Sometimes she made the cure for her neighbour's animals (cows, donkeys and sheep); 'You go out to the shed or ... the trailer and make it.'

She acquired this cure when she was a baby because a glove containing certain herbs was placed on her hand as she was baptised: 'You have to be christened with these herbs in your right hand ... and the picture of the Sacred Heart ... you put a wee mitten on the child's hand.' Nobody was aware of the exact herbs involved and they used the original baby glove each time there was a child baptised. Her two sisters were christened in this way also and they had the cure, as had her son and nephews; 'it's been carried on in the generations'. The cure had been in her family for more than a century. She started making it when she was about nine years old with the help of her grandmother; 'someone would come ... she might let me do it ... and she'd watch me'. She in turn taught her younger sisters how to make the cure.

This woman welcomed the steady flow of people who came to her home for the cure, often young people with sports injuries, local Gaelic players and soccer professionals from the large town nearby. Most people were strangers, primarily from the western counties and sometimes from other parts of Ireland. The cure had remained locally and when people returned looking for the grandmother, as they often did, they found the granddaughters. Her cure was deeply connected to her granny; 'for Granny's sake [she made it] ... to carry it on ... I know she would be so proud of us.' She had complete faith in her cure and believed it to have 'a great success rate ... It wouldn't live, if it didn't work.'

The cure was primarily a faith cure, with a vestige of the herbal healing tradition attached to it. I had interviewed her grandmother twenty years previously, and she told me that the herbs involved were robin-run-the-hedge (could be cleavers, large bindweed or ground ivy), goldenrod (used as an anti-inflammatory, and to heal wounds and sores), and a third yellow plant which she did not know the name of, but which she could point out in the field. Cleavers also have an anti-inflammatory affect, and in Mrs Grieve's English herbal, published in 1931, she stated that robin-run-the-hedge was a synonym for ground ivy and that the 'expressed juice may also be advantageously used for bruises'.

## Faith Healers

I met a healer (late sixties) who lived close to a lovely lake and woodland in north Roscommon. People were continually arriving at her house the two days of the week, Mondays and Thursdays, that she carried out her healing work; three visits were necessary to complete a cure. She told me with confidence that she had cured 'everything ... I think there's nothing I didn't come up against.' She listed some of the ailments that she had helped: Crohn's disease, Lyme disease, cancer, blood clots, vertigo, infertility, thrush, glaucoma, farmer's lung, kidney problems, venous ulcers and broken marriages.

Surprisingly, she said that depression was one of the biggest problems she dealt with. 'I had three different people today with depression ... they're tired, they lose their energy ... their strength ... they're in a tunnel without light, and my healing is prayer and when they see the prayer, they'll see the light, and they'll pull themselves out of that tunnel.' She explained, 'They come and tell me their problem ... they tell me their story ... and I bless them and we say the prayer together ... I help them as best I can.' She asked them to say the healing prayer, which consisted of one Our Father and three Hail Marys, every day.

Touch was an important part of her healing ritual too, but unlike most healers who use their hands, she touched people with her foot. 'I touch them ... I make the sign of the cross with the foot ... the healing, it's in the foot.' She would ask them to sit down and she put her right foot over the area of the body where the problem was. 'I know exactly when I leave my foot on a person what's wrong with them ... the knowledge just comes to me ... it's coming from God ... I'm just an agent for him.' She said that she had had this healing ability since she was a child and that she was born breech; 'I was born that way, I was born with it ... [the] healing.' She felt that people viewed her as special; they told her so and they gave her numerous gifts, often of a religious nature (holy pictures and rosary beads). She did not charge a fee, but she accepted money, a lot of which she donated to charity.

I interviewed a middle-aged woman who was a full-time healer in south Donegal; she was also a mother, gardener and musician. When I asked her how she would describe herself, she answered, 'I would say it's just a gift ... a great gift ... a gift that you're born with.' She told me that she had helped a variety of conditions, particularly skin problems: psoriasis, eczema and acne. Some people came to her with serious illness; 'I won't say I have the cure for that, but ... I could help them with maybe their peace of mind.'

She saw people by appointment in a quiet room in her home and she gave everyone as much time as they needed; they 'could be here half an hour or three quarters ... sometimes it takes longer ... especially for men ... to talk to you and get it off their chest'. The person sat at a table opposite her and she held their hands; 'I put my two hands around your two wrists ... it's hands-on healing.' She only touched their hands and she made the cure in the same way each time irrespective of the ailment.

Her left hand curled tightly around the person's right hand and in the person's left hand she placed three small envelopes, each containing three sweets. She prayed silently as she was holding their hands; this part of the ritual usually took ten minutes. Then gradually her left hand relaxed and the fingers unfurled. She always looked at the palm of her hand and she said there she saw 'a map of your body, it's like an insight into the body ... all the organs of the body ... you can see inflammation ... it would show up what really is wrong'. She believed that when her fingers opened, the problem that the person had passed from them, through her, and was taken away.

She directed people to eat three of the sweets that had been in their hand later that day and to say a prayer (any one they chose) when taking them. They then needed to eat three more sweets nine days later and the final three sweets following another nine days. This was one cure finished and they had to wait nine days before starting a second cure. She advised people to get three cures over a three-month period. 'I would recommend the third cure ... to clear it completely.' She described the sweets as 'the link ... there has to be a link between me and the person, and it has to be something they eat'.

There was an elderly woman who lived on a small farm in Leitrim, near the border with County Fermanagh and Northern Ireland. Her cure was called 'the power of prayer' and she thought it could be helpful to many ailments. To make the cure she touched the sick person and prayed for them. Using her left hand (she is a *ciotóg*, left-handed) she touched wherever they had the problem, three times, and as she was doing this, she said a blessing.

For nine days she prayed (one decade of the Rosary) for the person to either St Martin or St Anthony, whichever they preferred, while a special St Martin candle was burning: 'Every time you say the prayer, you light the candle.' She asked the individual who wanted the cure to light a candle as well and to pray for their recovery. They agreed on a time and then both parties prayed at the same hour in their respective homes for nine consecutive days. She believed these prayers were critical to the success of the cure, 'If they don't do it, it's no good; if they miss a day, it's broke, the chain is broke.'

This woman made her cure infrequently, but she felt it worked well and that 'after the nine days … if it's God's will, they're right'. She had this cure because she was born on Good Friday and christened on Easter Sunday. 'I got it through the priest … there's a little girl, he says, will have a cure the longest day she lives … I'm blessing this wee girl's hand, there's one in a thousand … born of a Good Friday.'

I think her cure was an interesting mixture of contemporary religious practice and traditional healing belief. In Catholicism a novena takes place over nine days, and it involves public and private prayer, often to a particular saint; in the past these community ceremonies were popular in Ireland. Robert Day wrote in 1888 (120 years before I interviewed this woman) about his encounter with Paddy the Doctor on a country lane near Crosshaven in Cork Harbour. He described the man as enjoying a 'well-earned reputation of being skilled in the practice of medicine … [and of using] simple extracts drawn from the herbarium of his native fields, and heather-grown cliffs'. When Day enquired as to how he had commenced his healing work, Paddy replied, 'I was born upon a Good Friday, and the priest said if I was christened between the first and second Mass on Easter Sunday I would be a wonderful doctor, and able to cure all diseases.' Padraic O'Farrell recalled in his book *Irish Customs*, that 'If a woman gave birth to a son on Good Friday, she usually asked that he be baptised with the newly blessed oils on Easter Sunday, something that would give the gift of healing.'

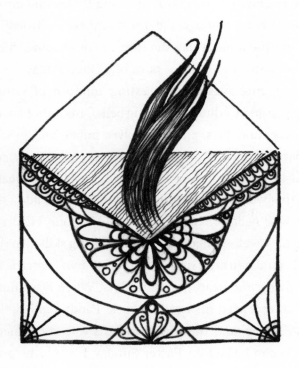

*An old man plucked hair from the cross on his donkey's back to make the asthma cure. This hair was placed in an envelope and under the child's pillow.*

# CHAPTER 5

## FAITH CURES

# Bleeds, Asthma, Hernias and Pains

### Bleeding

INTERVIEWED A FARMER AND cattle dealer, in his sixties, who lived on the banks of the Shannon in north Roscommon. He had a cure for bleeding or haemorrhaging, as he called it. His cure was a prayer, and it was used to stop bleeding in both humans and animals. He had been asked to help a variety of haemorrhages, including ones related to the nose, brain, threatened miscarriage, childbirth, operations, accidents and dehorned cattle.

The most amazing aspect of his cure was the numbers of people he made it for and the places they came from. This was an Irish cure with a truly international dimension. Over the thirty-three years that he had been making the cure he had received 'thousands of calls … six, eight, ten calls a day'. People phoned him from every part of Ireland and many from abroad, 'I get calls from ... all over the world ... England ... America ... New Zealand ... Canada', and even from the Congo and India. He speculated that these people probably had 'relatives in Ireland'.

As soon as it was requested, 'I say the [secret] prayer three times ... I ask for the cure for haemorrhaging and healing, and I ask, In the name of the Father, Son, and Holy Spirit each time.' He needed to have the name of the person with the bleed and he incorporated this into the cure. He also wanted to know what type of haemorrhage it was and if the person was in hospital. If the cure was for an animal, he asked the breed and colour, and the owner's name. 'I say it three times for ... the animal and the owner of the animal, I have to mention both.'

He never turned off his phone and often people called him during the night. He had had a mobile phone for twenty years, and consequently he and his cure were 'always accessible'. If he was watching a football match on the television and someone was injured and bleeding, he said the prayer for them. If he came upon a road accident or if an ambulance passed him when he was driving, he would make the cure.

He was given this cure (in about 1960) by a stranger, a man he met at a local cattle mart (sale). 'He just put it in my pocket ... he said to me that it might be useful ... it was written on a little bit of cardboard.' He looked at the card a few days later and was surprised to find that it was the cure for haemorrhaging. He put it away and forgot about the cure for sixteen years, until one day his baby boy had a severe nosebleed. 'In the midst of all the excitement ... I just thought, where's that prayer?' Even though he had moved house in the intervening years, 'I went upstairs and the first drawer I opened ... the prayer was sitting there ... [It was] a miracle!' 'I said it over him', and as he was saying the prayer the child's nosebleed stopped. This was the first of many, many cures, 'so I started to do it then ... I suppose I had belief.'

He continued to have complete faith in his cure and believed it to be hugely successful. Regularly he was asked to make the cure by relatives of people who were very sick in hospital or on their way there. 'I have known several people whose [brain] haemorrhaging had stopped before they got to Beaumont [hospital]', and operations were not needed. The only time he felt he couldn't help a bleed and that people may die, was if 'it's the Lord's way of bringing somebody'. He believed that God was the source of the healing in his cure. 'It's not me, I'll ask for the healing for the person, for the animal ... it's the Lord does the healing.' He was hugely positive about and respectful of his cure: 'It's extraordinary ... so, so important ... a gift ... why not share it ... especially if it could save a life.'

In the same county, but up in the hills, there was an elderly woman who also had a bleeding cure; she thought it was over one hundred years old. She too said a special, secret prayer, 'a prayer that my father left me before he died ... a very short prayer'. She usually said the prayer once. Occasionally, if the bleed did not stop, she would make the cure a second or even a third time, three days in a row. She told me of an old man locally who was bleeding badly and given only a few days to live. She made the cure three times for him and the bleeding stopped, and he lived ten more years. Another time, she met a neighbour in the hospital who was two months pregnant and haemorrhaging; 'I did it for her and she had her baby boy seven months later.' She preferred to see people in person and generally they came to her home. If this was not possible or they lived far away, they telephoned her and she would say the prayer for them. She felt that her cure worked equally well both ways.

I also spoke to a younger man (thirties) in rural south Monaghan who had a prayer cure for bleeding. He required four pieces of information about the person with the bleed: where they lived (town or townland), their age, hair colour and eye colour. Using these details, he created a mental image of the individual and focusing on this, he said the special cure prayer three times, then three Hail Marys, and to finish the cure he blessed himself. When I questioned him as to the significance of the number three, he said, 'The spiritual thing is three times ... everything was done in threes ... that's the magic in it.' His father gave him this cure and he had passed it on to others, while continuing to use it himself. 'I believe cures are for everybody ... God ... he wanted all people to be cured.'

## Asthma

There was a woman in her early forties, a mother and homemaker, who lived along the Wild Atlantic Way tourist trail in south Donegal. She had an asthma cure which she had been making for eight years and during that time she had helped almost seven hundred people, 'wee babies up to seventy-year-old men and women'. Those who wanted it either visited her or she posted the cure to them.

If they met face to face, she would lay her hands on them, one hand on their chest and the other on their back, 'directly opposite'. She held her hands like this for ten minutes, then she swapped around her hands and repeated the ritual. As she was touching the person she prayed silently and continuously; 'I say half on one side ... and half on the other ... there's a total of nineteen [prayers].' She made the cure in private; 'I put the kids out ... 'cos you have to concentrate on what you're doing.' She would experience heat when she was touching the person: 'I can feel heat pass from one side to the other ... I can feel it through the left hand.'

At the end of each visit, she would give the person a sealed envelope to take home with them. She told them to place the envelope 'between the pillow and the pillow slip, directly where you would lie ... near to the breathing'. It was vital that the envelope remained unopened; 'If you open the envelope the cure won't work,' she said. After three weeks she posted a second envelope to them, and following another three weeks she sent the third and final envelope of the cure, 'so they get a total of three altogether which they sleep on ... They always place the new one on top of the one that they have.' She would post the three envelopes to those who lived far away, such as in England, Germany and the USA. By the end of the nine-week period she believed most people were cured or their condition was much improved. If someone felt they needed a second cure, they had to wait nine weeks before getting it.

She had great respect for the traditional cures and it was partially because of this interest that she acquired her own cure. She had gone to Letterkenny in north Donegal in search of the asthma cure for a friend. The elderly woman who had it was unwell and she decided to give the cure to her. 'I walked into her house ... and she turned around to her husband and she says, "That's who I'm going to leave me cure to."' She told her how to make the cure and she 'passed' it to her; 'She put my left hand between her two hands and I could feel heat going from one side ... to the other.'

I interviewed a middle-aged man from a large town in the north-west who also had a faith cure for asthma. He was very secretive about his cure; however, he did say that he could only make it two days of the week, Tuesdays and Thursdays, and that it took about fifteen minutes to prepare. When somebody wanted the cure, they wrote to him or called to his house (he kept his phone number private). He made the cure for them, then posted it to their home or it could be collected. Often, he asked the person to write their name on an envelope, so that when the cure arrived, they would recognise it and open the letter.

In order to make the cure he had to know the name and age of the individual with the asthma. He gave them something to wear, and written instructions for what to do and what prayers to say. If it was a sick child, 'I hand the cure to its parents ... they open it, they put the cure on the child, they have to say the prayers.' He believed it was very important that the cure was not removed, rather that it was allowed to fall off and disappear of its own accord; 'If it ... disappears ... it's okay ... but if you take it off ... you have to start it again.'

He had inherited the cure from his mother thirteen years previously. She gave it to him three days before she died. Since then, he had made it for hundreds of people. He always asked them to let him know how they were feeling after the cure. His cure was well-known locally and farther afield in Ireland, the USA and England. In the three winter months prior to my conversation with him he had made it twenty-five times.

In a small town in north Leitrim there was a retired shopkeeper and he too had an asthma cure. He kept donkeys as pets and used the hair from the cross on their backs to make the cure. When it was requested, he clarified, 'I'll go out and I'll pluck the hair of the ass; you cannot cut it, you have to pluck it.' Ideally, he liked to take hairs from the intersection of the cross or close to their shoulders, as 'that's where Our Lady sat' on her journey to Bethlehem.

To make the cure, he would put a curly lock of the ass' hair into an envelope, seal it and write the initials of the person with the asthma on it. He instructed them to 'put it under your pillow ... leave it under the pillow ... as long as it takes'. If it got lost, he told them to come back for a second cure. He believed Our Lady was the source of the healing in this cure and he asked the person to say a prayer to her whenever they thought of the cure, 'any prayer ... the Hail Mary'.

He told me that many years earlier he had heard a woman talking about animals on a television programme (an Irish channel) and she had explained how this cure was made. The conversation left an impression on him and when he subsequently retired, 'I had time on me hands' and the donkeys, so 'I started at it.' He was enthusiastic about his cure, saying 'I take a delight in doing it.' I was interested to read, in Padraic O'Farrell's *Irish Folk Cures*, of the tradition of farmers taking a hair from the cross on a donkey's back and placing it on an animal's wound, and that 'any worm or moth alighting near it died'.

## Hiatus Hernia

I spoke to a man in his fifties who lived in east Leitrim, not far from the border with Cavan. He drove a school bus, had a small farm and a cure for hiatus hernia (when part of the stomach has moved up through the diaphragm opening into the chest cavity). He told me that the people who came to him had already been diagnosed by a doctor. He also said that for his cure to be successful, 'I think you have to believe in it ... most people that will come ... will have the belief, or they wouldn't have come to you in the first place.'

He wanted to keep the details of how he made his cure secret but he did tell me, 'I have prayers to say ... and I use a wee candle ... a glass ... a piece of bread', and that it only took 'a few minutes'. 'I don't talk to anyone about the cure' and he preferred that those receiving it did not either. The cure was made over three consecutive days, Thursdays and Mondays only, and the same ritual was repeated each day. His cure was unusual in that it had to be made before noon; 'that's the way it was told to me ... they normally come around eleven', a good time to catch him, after the school bus run and breakfast.

This was a cure that needed to be passed from woman to man, to woman. An old woman in County Cavan, a stranger, gave him the cure. He had gone to her with his late wife and mother to get the cure, 'and then she asked mum would I take the cure', and he did. He never saw this woman again, but when she died, he went to her wake; 'I wanted to touch her hand.' He remembered her family had a big welcome for him and that 'they were all wondering why did she pick me'. Every time he made the cure, he thought of this woman; 'I always think of her ... she'd be there in spirit.'

He had had his cure for ten years and made it for about a dozen people annually; more came in the autumn and winter, 'the back end of the year'. He believed that the healing comes from 'the prayers ... it's a faith cure'. He was a caring person and he reflected, 'I hope I'm doing someone good ... I'm doing it for no reward ... I get satisfaction if I can [help].' This man had great faith in the traditional cures and felt they were still popular in his locality. 'I believe in cures ... it's a good thing ... there's a reason for them.'

There was a man in Monaghan, a lorry driver, who had a similar cure for hiatus hernia; I mentioned him earlier in relation to his bleeding cure. He used a glass, a small candle and a large, copper penny to make the cure. Before he started, he explained the procedure to the person to reassure and relax them. He asked them to lie down and to pull up their shirt so that he could place the coin on their skin, 'under the breastbone'. He put a lighted candle on top of the penny and covered both with a glass. 'You give it a slight twist to make the glass stick ... it cuts out the air ... it'll suck the skin up into the glass ... about half an inch ... they get a sensation ... of pulling into the glass.' He would then remove the glass and penny, relight the candle, and repeat the ritual twice more, three times in total. As he was doing the procedure, he asked the person to pray silently, any prayer of their choice, and he said some prayers.

People had to pay him three visits (at his house) to complete this cure, on three consecutive days, so that the ritual with the candle was performed nine times altogether. He could make the cure any time, but he tended to see people on Monday, Tuesday and Wednesday nights and to give each person an appointment, 'every fifteen minutes'. Also, for practical and privacy reasons he shared this cure with his wife, so that she could 'do women ... I do the men.'

For the cure to work he felt strongly that people must believe in it; 'they have to have some sort of a belief in it ... or there's no point in coming ... I'm doing my bit 100 per cent all the time.' He understood that the source of the healing was God; 'It's God energy ... you're just a channel ... allowing the energy to channel through you ... into the person.'

I interviewed a grandmother in the midlands who had this cure too; she referred to it as the cure for the breastbone. The cure had been passed down through the women in her family, from her grandmother, to her mother, to her. In time, she hoped to give it to one of her daughters. She had been making the cure for over twenty years, but had had it for much longer. For a long while, she was not using it because she was busy rearing her family. One day she went to a faith healer looking for help with her asthma, and they told her that she had a cure and that she should use it; a fortnight later someone came looking for it.

Dr Logan wrote that the hiatus hernia cure was also known as 'the spoon of the chest (cléithín)'. Dr Fleetwood recalled that, 'Cupping was practised by the early Irish leeches [physicians] ... This operation in which a vacuum is created over a painful skin area is seldom employed nowadays, although at times it may give great relief without the use of drugs.'

## Colic

Close to a large town in the north-west a Traveller man lived on a halting site with his young family. He had a cure for colic and primarily helped babies, 'from about two weeks, onwards to three or four months'. To make the cure, he held a black bootlace over the child's stomach. He created a large loop and tied a loose knot at the top of it, as he silently said a prayer. He created a second large loop above the first one and this he also closed with a loose knot. Taking one end of the lace, he wove it through the two loops. To finish the ritual, he pulled taut both ends of the lace to open it out straight so that it was free of knots.

This quick procedure was performed three times and repeated for three days, nine times in total. He had adapted his cure; in the past it was only made on Mondays and Thursdays, but when I interviewed him he would start it on whatever day the baby was first brought to him. The second and third visits took place on the following Monday and Thursday, or vice versa. He believed it was essential to the success of the cure that he performed the ritual over the child for three days.

This man had had his cure for five years, and in that time he had become well-known for it and had helped 'five or six hundred people'. The numbers looking for the cure varied from week to week; 'you could have two one week ... or twelve'. The people were from the west (Galway, Roscommon and Sligo), from Athlone, and some came from Dublin. He kept the bootlace in his wallet so that it was always to hand if needed. He would not accept money for his cure; 'to take money for it ... breaks the cure; it won't work,' he asserted. But he did accept gifts, often biscuits or chocolate for his children, and he believed that this practice of giving something in return for the cure was part of the cure.

I spoke to a man living on a small farm in south Leitrim who had a colic cure too. He made it daily and helped animals (cattle and horses) as well as people; I had heard about him from a vet. He was elderly and in poor health so his wife assisted him. When the cure was requested, she would tie and untangle two knots in a brown shoelace as he said the secret prayers. This ritual was carried out three times, on one day only, and it took just a few minutes to complete. The sick child did not have to be physically present, and most people telephoned and asked for the cure. They phoned from all over Ireland, and from the USA and Canada. He liked to know 'the name of the child, where she is living ... you think of the child'.

He told me of two traditions that were attached to this cure; he could not accept money for it, and someone could not ask for the cure to be passed to them. Nearly forty years previously a neighbouring woman had given it to him. He had arranged that the cure would remain in the family; it would go to his son.

In rural south Sligo there was a man who was very interested in the traditional cures and thought they had remained strong in his area. He made three cures, including one for colic. His daughter had given him this cure six years earlier because she was moving to England. She said, 'Dad, I better give you this, because people will still be calling and I wouldn't want them to be turned away.' A friend in primary school, a Traveller boy, had given her the cure.

The procedure involved making and untying a knot nine times on a length (about 30 cm) of ordinary string, while saying three prayers repeatedly, Our Father, Hail Mary and Glory Be. He believed that 'the knot is to represent the knot in the [child's] gut and the removal of the knot is to represent the removal of the knot in the gut'. Some people preferred to bring their baby to him, but more often they phoned him and he made the cure straight away.

This man had complete belief in his cures, but for the colic cure he felt that those receiving it may not have faith in it, yet it would still work; 'the child doesn't know you're doing it ... or the horse!' He believed that someone who has a cure is blessed, that should always make it when asked, and 'if you are not going to use it ... you should pass it on to somebody else'.

O'Farrell wrote of this cure; it was thought that the colic was 'caught' by the knot, and that it 'fell' to the bottom of the string and was taken away, also, that 'Some communities called the practice *sníomh na péiste* (worm or reptile's twist).' Phil Cronin investigated traditional cures in County Mayo and in 2002 she published a booklet based on her research. She recorded the colic cure, which involved the intricate knotting of a piece of twine, as *snaidhm péiste* (worm knot).

## Sciatica

I interviewed an eighty-year-old man who lived at the edge of a County Roscommon town; he had a popular cure for sciatica. This cure involved quite a challenging ritual. Those who wanted the cure had to visit him three times and each time they had to bring water to him. But it was a specific type of water that was required; it must be water that had been taken from a flowing river between two counties. The water could only be collected at night-time and it was used in the making of the cure the following day. 'You have to lift water between any two counties ... lifted before sunrise and used before sunset ... if the sun has risen it's no use.' In addition, he stipulated that it should not be collected before 'a quarter to two in the morning'.

He felt the safest way to get this water was to tie a string to a bottle and to drop it into a river from a bridge. To people living in that area, he recommended the bridge across the Shannon at Lanesborough, between Counties Roscommon and Longford. Those availing of the cure could collect the water personally or ask someone to do this task on their behalf. He said that only a small amount of water was needed in the bottle, 'half an inch ... that's plenty', but that fresh water must be brought along to each of the three visits: 'It has to be lifted the three turns,' he insisted.

The person who wanted the cure would come to his home before sunset, having acquired the water the previous night. He would put the water in a little bowl, dip his right index finger in it and rub it on the areas affected by the sciatica: 'the water must be touched to [the skin] wherever you have the pain'. As he was doing this, he asked the person to say fifteen prayers, five Our Fathers, five Hail Marys and five Glory Bes. He also prayed silently and kept these prayers secret, though he did say 'there's a lot of Latin in it'.

He made the cure on Mondays, Thursdays and Saturdays, and repeated the same ritual each day. He liked people to finish it within one week: 'If they fail to come one day, they can wait for that day the following week ... but that's prolonging [the cure].' He usually asked people to come to him at lunchtime and he could see up to ten people in that hour. Most of them were strangers and many had travelled long distances, including from Cork and Kerry. He thought that almost everyone had already been with a doctor.

This man believed his cure to have a high success rate and that 'one month from the day they finish there should not be any pain'. He always asked people to contact him four weeks after the cure to let him know the outcome, if they have 'slight pain, bad pain or no pain'. He felt this was an important aspect of the cure and that the pain could possibly return if he did not hear from them. He had been making this cure for almost forty years. His mother had it before him; she received it from his grandfather. He hoped to pass it to his daughter; 'it has to go back to a woman'. He was a kind man and he said, 'If I stopped [giving the cure] ... how many would I leave suffering ... when I know I can do good for someone. I like doing it.'

## Bell's Palsy

There was a man living in the Armagh countryside, near the border with the Republic and County Monaghan, who told me that the cures are 'still very popular' and that in his vicinity 'there's lots of people with charms for different things'. He was fifty years old, friendly and articulate, the director of a beautiful, old hotel, and he had a Bell's palsy cure. He said that this problem was caused by a trapped nerve in the face (one side of the face droops) and that his cure was used to help damaged nerves in other parts of the body as well, such as the neck, shoulder, back and wrist.

If the problem was with the face, he commenced the cure by placing his hands there. He then moved his hands (with the thumbs overlapped and his palms touching the clothes) slowly down the person's body and out along their arm, as if drawing the ailment away. He did this nine times while saying a special prayer each time. If the trapped nerve was in the neck, he explained, 'you start off at the neck by laying on of hands, you travel down the back and then out into one or other leg, and down to the ground; you are taking it out ... [You] must move down.' As he was making the cure people often experienced 'a tingling sensation', others felt heat from his hands, and some a 'slight pain ... They'll feel it moving; that's a good sign.'

He recited the cure prayer silently as he was touching the person. He described it less as a prayer and more as words that Jesus would have spoken. 'The prayer that I say goes back to Our Lord ... it's words that Our Lord would have said while ... healing someone ... you can never tell anyone those words because that breaks the cure.' To complete the cure people had to visit him three times, and they had the laying on of hands and prayer ritual repeated nine times each visit. 'My charm is done on three visits, three days in between, so that's nine days [from start to finish].'

He believed that God was the source of the healing. He described himself as a channel for the 'power ... coming from Our Lord Jesus ... God gave his son the power to heal, and by me laying on my hands that power goes through me.' He elaborated by saying his cure is 'a gift that's been given to you to use ... you have to use that power correctly ... If I stop it, I lose it and it's lost forever.' He started making this cure when he was a teenager and was given it by his mother. 'It comes through our family ... my grandfather ... my mother ... it goes from male to female each generation.' He intended to give it to his eldest daughter and in time he hoped her son would inherit it. He said, 'Once I tell my daughter those words, then she has to use it, I can't use it.'

He told me that the cure had had a good effect on his life and that it helped to be 'a people person, you have to enjoy meeting people ... to be confident with them ... easy enough about them coming into your home'. This man was clear in his understanding of the cure, stating that 'with my charm I can't advertise it, I can't charge for it, and I can't refuse it'. He was a generous person; for him his cure was 'never a chore ... I meet some very nice people ... I will do the charm for anyone who asks.'

## Shingles

I spoke to a man in his sixties from a small town in north Donegal. He was a bus driver, butcher and fiddler, and had a well-known shingles cure. How he made his cure was a secret, but it involved prayer and touch. He would briefly touch the area where the shingles were with something, which he kept wrapped in a handkerchief, and as he was doing this, he prayed. He liked to be quiet and to concentrate when he was making the cure. He asked the person getting the cure to be silent and to close their eyes, so that they would not see what was in his hand.

The cure ritual was quick and people visited him once. Some came back for a second cure one week or ten days later. They normally called to his house and he made it in the hallway or sitting room. He worked for many years in a local butcher's shop and people were always dropping in there for the cure. He had had this cure for nearly half a century and as the years passed it grew in popularity; on average he made it twice a week. He was always expecting someone and when I rang his doorbell, he thought I had come for the cure.

This man was a good listener and people liked to talk to him about their shingles, their lives and their problems. From his years of experience with this condition he believed shingles could be caused by stress, trauma and bereavement. People got it at times when they were vulnerable and their energy levels were low. I asked him what he felt was the source of the healing in his cure and he replied that it could be psychological. He felt that those receiving his cure must believe in it for it to work and that they did believe in it because they came for it. He also thought that we all have an ability to fight illness and to cure ourselves.

# Eyes

I met a quiet-spoken, middle-aged farmer in south Sligo who had a faith cure for 'the mote in the eye'. A mote, he said, was any foreign body in the eye, such as dust or glass. Mote is defined as a tiny spec in the dictionary. People usually telephoned and asked him to make the cure. To do this he had to have two pieces of information about the injured person, their name and the general area where they lived.

He made the cure as soon as possible after the phone call. 'I have to go into a private place' and 'I say the prayers and do the cure ... but I cannot tell you exactly what I do.' He believed the prayers were 'the main part of the cure' and he said them every day, whether he was making a cure or not, 'to keep the cure [alive]'. If people called to his house looking for the cure, he invited them in to 'sit down, and I go away in privacy and do the cure'.

He felt that his cure was quite effective; it normally worked quickly and the foreign body 'will come out of the eye ... some people have got nearly instant relief, more the following morning'. He knew that most of those who got his cure have been to a doctor first, but with little success; 'I've got phone calls from people in Casualty [hospital].' He recommended medical attention if the eye injury was very bad or slow to heal. This man thought the best approach was often both to see a doctor and to get his cure.

There was another farmer in the same county with a similar cure. His cure, which took about five minutes to make, involved secret prayers and a 'couple of saucers of water'. 'I was told not to tell [the procedure] by the old lady,' he clarified. Once he had received the request for the cure, generally by phone, he made it in a quiet room. He never saw anything in the saucers of water when he was making the cure, though he understood that others with this cure did.

He made his cure any day of the week 'between sunrise and sunset'. Having said this, if someone phoned after dark looking for the cure he would oblige, but he would also make it a second time for the person the following morning. Twenty-six years earlier he was given the cure by an elderly neighbour, a woman his wife had cared for. It had to be passed from woman to man, to woman, and when he feels the time is right, he will give it to one of the younger women in his family.

I had a conversation with a woman who lived on the west Sligo coastline and who made a comparable cure. She mainly helped people who got dirt in their eye or bits of metal when welding. The injured person did not have to come to her, but she needed to know their name. She took a drink of water and held it in her mouth as she silently said a secret prayer, five times. Then she spat the water on to a saucer and repeated this ritual twice more.

She told me that often she would see 'dirt' in the water that she had spat out and this she believed was the particle that was causing the eye problem. She had had the cure for more than twenty years and inherited it from her mother. When I enquired about this cure in a pub in the nearby surfing village, the Australian barman told me that he had heard great reports about this woman and her cure.

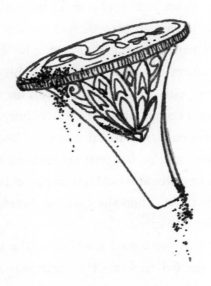

*One seventh son used a gold wedding ring to make the sign of the cross on the ringworm; he dipped the ring in earth first.*

# CHAPTER 6

# Seventh Daughters and Sons

T HE TRADITION OF THE SEVENTH daughter or son having healing power has been very strong in Ireland. If seven girls or seven boys are born consecutively in a family, the seventh child will be able to heal ringworm and sometimes other conditions. It will not work, for example, if there are seven girls, but a boy is born in between them. Stillborn babies are counted, so if seven boys are born and one of them has died at birth, the seventh child will still have the cure. I interviewed nine people who have this special healing status. All of them cure ringworm which is the ailment seventh daughters and sons are traditionally linked to. One woman was also able to get rid of warts, another woman helped a variety of skin problems, and two men were full-time faith healers; these healers dealt with a wide range of illnesses.

Ringworm, or tinea, is a fungal skin infection which forms a red, itchy rash, usually in the shape of a ring, expanding outwards as it heals centrally. It affects many parts of the body, is highly contagious, and can be passed from animals to humans. Some of the seventh daughters and sons I talked to cure animals, generally horses, of ringworm, using the same procedure as they would for a person.

I came across a reference to seventh daughters and sons in Welsh folk medicine. Anne Jones conducted research there in the late 1970s, and she had found that 'the seventh son or seventh daughter in a direct line of descent that was totally male or female' possessed a healing gift. David Hoffman recorded an old cure for warts in Wales too, which was to wash them with the water from a font in which a seventh son had been baptised. Lady Wilde wrote in 1888 that, 'When a seventh son is born, if an earth-worm is put into the infant's hand and kept there till it dies, the child will have power to charm away all diseases.' Dr Logan has written 'it would seem that the ancient Irish believed that worms caused certain diseases', and that in Anglo-Saxon 'the word "wyrm" may mean a worm, an insect, a snake or a dragon'. I suspect that the 'worm' may be a covert representation of the pagan goddess, who was suppressed and demonised as the patriarchal Christian religion took control of Ireland.

I spoke to a woman in her early twenties who was a seventh daughter with a cure for ringworm. She worked as a secondary-school teacher, and had grown up on a small farm in County Sligo. Her parents knew of the tradition of the seventh daughter having this cure and they tested her with a worm when she was a baby. 'If you get an earthworm, put it in the child's hand and put the other hand over ... that's how you know you have the cure ... the worm died in my hand,' she explained. When I spoke to her, it was still the case that if she put a worm in her hand the same thing happened: 'the minute it goes on my hand it struggles' and it will die within three to four minutes. Many of the seventh daughters and sons that I interviewed told me a similar story.

She described how she made her cure as a simple procedure. 'I just put both my hands ... on it [the ringworm] ... put my right hand on it for at least one to two minutes, and then swap over and put my left hand on it for one to two minutes, and that's it.' For a very large affected area, she would move both hands over it at the same time. 'I can talk throughout ... the process ... I try and make them feel comfortable.' Occasionally, she felt a burning sensation in the centre of her hand, especially if the ringworm had not been there long; 'If it's new, it's fresh, it can be getting hotter.' The client would feel nothing. I asked her about the word 'client' and she said that she was unsure of what to call the people who came for her cure and that this was the term she eventually settled on.

Those who wanted the cure visited her on three separate days, and tradition stipulated that these were Mondays and Thursdays. However, she was flexible and if people could not come on the specified days, she would see them on a different one. If the ringworm had been there for three weeks or more, they might have had to come to her four or five times. 'The fresher it is, the sooner you come, the sooner you get rid of it,' she said. Following the first healing session the condition would often get very itchy, but by the second visit the itch had generally subsided, and at the third visit the ringworm was usually disappearing.

Even though ringworm is contagious, she and her family members had never contracted it. She felt that her cure in some way protected her from this; 'I would never be conscious of getting it myself ... [I am] so safeguarded against it.' She told me that she started making the cure as a baby with the help of her parents and that it was an ever-present part of their family life. They were all involved in her cure: 'without them I wouldn't have the cure ... without my sisters I wouldn't be a seventh sister'. As an adolescent she became quite self-conscious and often wondered about her cure; 'Am I weird? I'm not like ordinary teenagers.' As an adult she was more accepting: 'it's just something I live with now'.

There was a woman living in a large town in the midlands; she was in her thirties and the mother of four young children. She was also a seventh daughter and could cure warts as well as ringworm. I had known this woman since she was a child as her grandmother's house was close to my family home and she often came on holidays there. Her mother was present on the day of this interview and contributed to the conversation. They told me that the first time she used her cure (at age four) was to heal my little sister of severe ringworm on her arms and legs. My mother, who had great faith in the traditional cures, had asked would the child make the cure; she did and it worked very well.

She was born (1974) in the nursing home of a County Longford town and a nun working there asked could the baby be tested with a worm. So, when she was just three days old a worm was put in her right hand, and her parents watched as it stopped wriggling and died. 'We all witnessed this,' her mother recalled. As a child, she often made her cure in school (at lunchtime) for people who called by looking for it, or in the evenings at her home.

Her cure remained popular and in recent years she made it more for warts than ringworm. She used the same ritual for both cures. 'I just make the sign of the cross on the parts that has the ringworm or warts and I say prayers.' She could say any prayer she liked, usually a few Hail Marys and Our Fathers. She always used her right hand and as she was saying the prayers, she stroked the warts/ringworm repeatedly. It was a quick procedure, taking just five minutes, but it had to be repeated on two other days (Thursdays and Mondays). Regularly she felt heat when she made her cure. 'I would get a burning sensation in my hands ... I'd have to put cold water on them ... when the burning sensation came first [in childhood] it frightened me.'

I interviewed an eighty-six-year-old woman who lived on a farm in Mayo, and enjoyed tending to her hens and flowers. She was a mother, a grandmother and a seventh daughter. There were nine children in her family, and 'I was the youngest daughter,' she remembered. She cured ringworm as well as other skin problems, including eczema, psoriasis and shingles. She told me that there were two types of ringworm – 'there's a male and a female' – but that did not affect her ability to cure them.

She always made her cure the same way, irrespective of the skin disorder. She would pray silently; 'I just say a couple of prayers, any prayer at all ... I pray that they'll be alright' and she touched the person with her right hand on the skin where the problem was, 'just one spot'. She had to touch the person three times and each time after she touched them, she touched the ground. When I spoke with her she was elderly and no longer knelt to touch the floor; however, she said, 'I can rub me hand anywhere instead of the ground ... three times.' I believe that she touched the ground (or the wall) to 'transfer' the ailment into it.

Like the other seventh daughters, she repeated this ritual for three days. 'You have to come three times ... Mondays and Thursdays [consecutive] ... if they break it, they have to start again.' After the person had left, she would think of them; 'I still pray for them, when they're finished ... I'd be praying for them six months after.' She, like most people with cures, did not question or analyse her cure; she just accepted and made it. When I asked her was there any secret attached to her cure she said, 'No ... [and] nobody ever asked me how I did it, [before you!]'

While they were receiving the cure and until the problem fully cleared, she requested that the person not drink alcohol or wet the affected area, and to wear white clothing next to it, which she thought would be 'cleaner' against the skin. She did not feel heat when she put her hand on someone, but she said they would often say that they did; 'that shows that it's working ... They feel heat or they may feel some sort of tingling going through them.' Her cure was very popular; 'hundreds ... I do have seven and eight here many a day ... they never stop [coming]'. She helped all sorts of people, 'lovely people' she recalled, especially the children. She told me that her cure was 'a gift', and 'while there's breath in me', she would keep making it. 'I love helping people ... I'd be as interested in them getting better, as they would themselves.'

I had a thought-provoking conversation with a middle-aged man from a big town in the north-west. This man was well-read and articulate, and he was a seventh son. He rarely made his cure now, but as a child he cured hundreds of people of ringworm. His family and community had complete faith in his ability to heal; he remembered himself as 'a four-year-old surrounded by people who totally believe what they are about to experience'. His father would regularly accompany him when he made the cure. 'We'd go into the sitting room ... you step into a "space" ... it's almost as if I took a breath ... and in that "space" there was no failure ... no hesitation ... everyone was quiet and you just done it.' He also said that in his youth he found it difficult being different to other children.

He described the way in which he cured ringworm. 'I touch it with my hand, in the name of the Father, the Son, and the Holy Spirit, Amen.' He would touch and withdraw his hand three times as he said this blessing, touching the ringworm to coincide with the words Father, Son and Holy Spirit. Again, the cure took place over three days, but it did not matter which three days, so long as they were in a row. Usually, by the second visit the ringworm had started to dry up and to diminish. Often, he felt a tingling sensation and heat in his hand when he made the cure, or even when he thought or talked about it.

There was a man in his thirties, a father of young children, and a breeder and trainer of horses. He lived in a village in east Sligo and he too was a seventh son with a ringworm cure. He grew up in Dublin, but his parents were from rural Ireland and were aware of the seventh son healing tradition. He seldom made his cure when he lived in the city; however, when he moved to the countryside ten years before I spoke to him, local people discovered that he was a seventh son and started asking him for the cure. 'It was kind of word of mouth.'

He believed faith in his cure was crucial to its success. He recalled a man who was badly affected by ringworm; this man was an employee and initially he was sceptical of the cure. 'He used to giggle when I was blessing him; he wouldn't take it seriously ... it kept getting worse.' One day they were in Dublin together, 'I brought him to the church that I was baptised in, blessed him, and it was gone in two days ... there wasn't a mark on his arm.' He said that the young man had taken the cure seriously this time and was healed.

This man used holy water as part of the cure ritual, and I met another seventh son who used a gold wedding ring. He dipped the ring in earth, then made the sign of the cross with it on the inflamed skin, three times, ensuring that the ring was always in contact with the skin, and he silently said a blessing each time. To finish the cure, he asked the person to bless themselves. This procedure was repeated on three consecutive days.

He welcomed all those who arrived at his door and sometimes his wife offered them a cup of tea. But he said that many did not delay and that they could be embarrassed, as 'people get ringworm in awkward places'. For this reason or if he was healing children, he would insist that his wife was present when he was giving the cure. He started making his cure as a boy, having been shown how to do it by his mother and grandmother. Over a sixty-year period he had cured thousands of people of ringworm in the port town in the north-west where he lived.

I also interviewed a man in his forties from rural Sligo. He was married with children, worked as a mechanic and was a seventh son. He liked to make his cure for ringworm in a quiet, private place, so that he could concentrate on what he was doing. 'I wouldn't talk to them ... you are putting all your energy into it ... you are thinking totally about that.' One of the traditions attached to his cure was that it should be made 'before sunset' and he always adhered to this as a child. As an adult, for practical reasons, he occasionally made his cure after sunset with no apparent effect on the success of the cure. 'I would do it in the dark ... I'd be home late ... it does work.' This man thought that his cure was 'a gift from God'. He would not accept money for it and he felt that if he were to, he might lose his cure; 'you don't charge for a gift ... I'd be afraid it wouldn't work ... you're doing it out of goodness of heart.'

In south Leitrim I spoke to a man who was a full-time faith healer because he was born a seventh son. Initially he cured ringworm, warts and eczema, and he believed his success rate as a child healer was 'very close on 100 per cent'. Interestingly, he said it was easier to heal as a child; 'nobody doubted the integrity of the child healer. They had great trust in them. There was no issue with commercialism.' But as he grew older the element of trust lessened; 'adulthood brings its own problems ... People are afraid to be let down ... to be taken in by someone.' By the time he turned eighteen his reputation as a healer was firmly established and he made a conscious decision to focus on this aspect of his life.

For the next twenty years his work as a faith healer expanded, and he became widely known and respected. He told me that he had had success with many health concerns, such as psoriasis, shingles, asthma, ulcers, arthritis, back pain, tumours and depression. He was brought to England and the USA to help people who were usually of 'Irish descent'. Thousands of people turned to him for assistance. 'I could see a few hundred people a week ... it varies ... I've never had an idle day in thirty-nine years.' All ages and all types of people came to him. Some of them were religious, some spiritual and some atheists; 'they interpret it [the healing] accordingly ... to suit their own needs'. He charged a modest fee for each consultation and kept paper records. 'I keep a log of each case ... the name, address, what the condition was ... I keep [financial] accounts.'

In the past his cure was made on Mondays and Thursdays; then he started to see people at his home, or a hotel 'clinic' in some large town other days. Those looking for a cure would visit him three times; he elaborated by saying, 'Three consultations [are] consistent with the Trinity ... Father, Son, and Holy Spirit.' People waited in his sitting room and then one by one they entered his office, sat down and told him their problem; 'it's a personal thing between two people ... Everyone is afforded whatever amount of time is needed ... five minutes to an hour.' He was a relaxed man and gave each person his full attention. 'Every new case is special; it's the same as starting again as a healer ... It's not supposed to be easy.'

He would lay his hands on the person, keeping them for a short while on the area where the problem was located, and as he was doing this he would pray silently. He said that a transfer of 'healing energy' took place between him and the person he was helping. He would ask people if they felt heat or energy coming from his hands, and if they did, he took this as a good sign. He thought that many of the people who came to him had already been with a doctor. They had got 'conventional treatment and found it's not helping' so they tried him, 'as a last resort'.

It was important that those who came to him trusted him; 'with me, people need to have ... trust ... specifically [trust] in the gift of healing'. Some people looked for a cure 'to please someone else' but this was not helpful as the person had to want to be healed; 'there has to be a focus ... "Belief" is an important aspect of the cure.' He was an insightful man who expressed his thoughts on healing clearly. 'It's about the psychological ... as well as the physical and spiritual ... there's three levels of healing.' He felt that stress is 'one of the main sources of ill health'. He believed too that some 'people deny themselves the right to recover', that they can be sceptical and doubtful, and that they can over focus on the illness (the negative) and under focus on the healing (the positive).

This man understood that he, as a healer, must remain humble and not view himself as special, because 'that specialness can create a barrier or a blockage'. He felt that his healing ability was 'a God-given gift ... it's a greater force at work'. When I asked him why he healed, he replied, 'because it works' and he told me that he would only stop healing 'when the last knock comes to the door'. 'I enjoy it immensely

… I have met some fabulous people … I love every time the door opens and someone new walks in.'

There was another well-known faith healer living in south Leitrim; I interviewed him when he was eighty-seven and in good health. He confidently said, 'I have the cure for everything' and proceeded to list a variety of ailments that he had helped: asthma, diabetes, psoriasis, haemorrhages, shingles and cancer. He had his cure because he was a seventh son, but did not start using it until he was in his thirties. His first cure was of a child with eczema. The girl's grandmother, his former teacher, had faith in his ability to heal; 'you have a cure she says, and if you say a prayer … for that child, I believe she'll get well'. She did, and that was the start of his healing 'career'.

His cure entailed talking and listening to the person, blessing them with holy water, laying on of hands and prayer. 'You have to listen to people … they tell me what's wrong with them … I don't believe I'd be able to cure them if I didn't listen to them right,' he stressed. He blessed everyone with holy water on their forehead, using his thumb. Then he placed his hands on the seated person's head as he said (secret) prayers silently, 'about five or six minutes I'd be praying … I do pray … that they'll get well.' When 'I put me hands on their head … they feel shocking [very] relaxed, and they tell me often … "I was nearly asleep"; that's the best sign in the world.' He felt no heat but he said, 'they feel a heat in me hands'.

His healing reputation had stretched to every corner of Ireland and as a younger man people came to his home daily in search of cures. As an older man he saw them in a back room of the local village pub, two days per week, for a few hours. He limited the numbers, and everyone phoned in advance and was given an appointment time. Often his schedule would run late; 'You have to talk to people,' he explained, and the *bean an tí* (landlady) would shout to him to hurry up, that there was a queue waiting downstairs! People travelled long distances, so he had adapted his cure and asked them to come just once. 'I only bring them once ... faith healers as a rule brings them three times, but I don't ... it's too far.'

I found him to be a gentle and caring person. He told me that many people came to him with depression. 'I had a young woman today ... she cried and cried ... that's an awful thing, depression.' He philosophically said that years ago 'there was no money in this country and the people were far happier'. He did not charge for his healing work but he did accept money; 'some people give money ... I never ask ... it doesn't matter whether they have money [or not] ... I do the same thing for them.'

This man was making his cure for more than fifty years and he had helped thousands of people. Even though he was very elderly, he said, 'I never feel one bit tired [when healing] ... there's a God in Heaven ... and he has something to do with it ... that's why I do it ... and I'll continue while I'm alive.' During the writing of this book, he died, and the online death notice described him as a faith healer. I attended his funeral as did hundreds of other people whom he had cured or touched in some way over his many years of healing.

I visited a woman in north Mayo whose late husband was a seventh son; he had cured ringworm, shingles and cowpox. She made the cure occasionally after his death and had found that it still worked. Using his unwashed pyjamas, she performed the same ritual as he had, touching the floor three times with her hand, blessing herself once, and then rubbing the skin which was affected with his clothing. Like numerous other cures, this one took place over three days. She told me that her husband had regularly made his cure on to a piece of cloth, usually a white handkerchief, and that he had posted these 'cure cloths' around the world, to England, the USA, New Zealand and Australia.

Human touch can be powerful, positive and healing. Kaptchuk and Croucher investigated hand-healing in the 1980s and they cited scientific research from McGill University, Montréal, which found that, 'In a series of ingenious controlled experiments wounded mice healed more quickly and barley seeds grew faster' when a man with a healing reputation laid his hands on them.

Dr Una Kroll explored the meaning of disease, healing and wholeness in her book, *In Touch with Healing*. Disease she broadly defined as 'an absence of ease … that state which alerts us to our need of healing' and she highlighted the importance of an 'increased understanding of the connection between stress and physical disease'. With regard to the laying on of hands, Kroll feels that some healers can discern through their hands where the problem lies and what is causing it. 'The hands and the brain seem to be deeply in tune with each other.' She also believes that the healer can focus energy in their hands and can transmit this energy to the person they are touching. 'The recipient often feels a considerable amount of warmth … the donor's energy seems to release energy within the recipient … these healing energies somehow reinforce the energies and rhythms in all of us.'

# CHAPTER 7

## HERBAL CURES

# Cancer, Shingles, Jaundice, Gallstones and Skin

I N THE FOREWORD TO JOSÉ JAÉN'S *Handbook of Canary Folk Medicine*, botanist David Bramwell has written that, 'Medicinal plants began to be used more than 5,000 years ago ... their use in medicine has been practised in every human culture in history.' Hippocrates (known as the Father of Medicine) 'wrote more than 400 remedies based on plants'. The World Health Organization's *Traditional Medicines Strategy 2014–2023* states that for many people today, 'Across the world, traditional medicine is either the mainstay of health care delivery or serves as a complement to it', particularly in economically poor African and Asian countries. 'The strategy aims to support Member States in developing proactive policies ... that will strengthen the role traditional medicine plays in keeping populations healthy'.

The 2019 United Nations' (UN) Global Assessment Report on

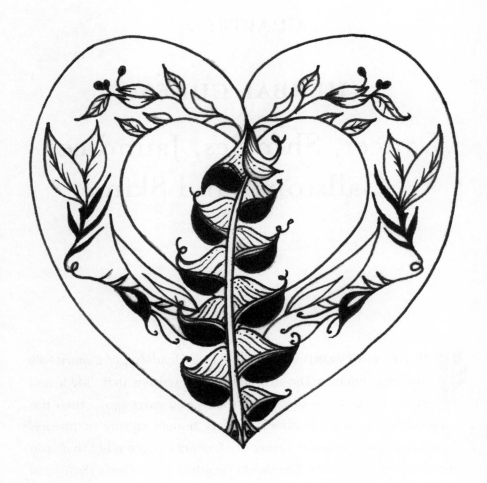

*The foxglove gives us digitalis, which is used to treat heart failure.*

Biodiversity, highlighted that 'an estimated 4 billion people rely primarily on natural medicines for their health care and some 70 per cent of drugs used for cancer are natural or are synthetic products inspired by nature'. Well-known medicines that are of plant origin include quinine (from cinchona bark), aspirin (from willow bark) and morphine (from opium poppy). When walking in the woods a few years ago with a cardiologist friend, he pointed to a beautiful foxglove and said that he had prescribed it the previous week; digitalis is extracted from the leaves, and used to treat heart failure and to control heart rate.

Worldwide, the pharmaceutical industry is more likely to investigate plants with a healing reputation and if found to be useful to isolate their active compounds. In contrast herbalism tends to use the whole plant or parts of it, which may mean that the herb acts more slowly and gently on the body, and side effects may be less likely. Thomas Bartram writes in his *Encyclopedia of Herbal Medicine*, that 'Herbalism is a science in its own right … It offers healing properties that favourably influence chemical change, combat stress, build up resistance to infection and promote vitality.' A word of warning though, herbs may be natural, wild and free, but care must be exercised when identifying and collecting them, as some plants are highly poisonous.

The use of plant life for healing purposes was widespread in Ireland up to the middle of the twentieth century, as verified by the multitude of herbal cures (for people and animals) documented in The Schools' Collection 1937–39. In the past many Irish people lived close to the land and nature, and over the centuries an understanding of plants and their medicinal qualities had been accumulated, through experimentation, and the sharing of knowledge orally within families and communities. The observation of what sick animals ate would have been useful too as they seemed to know instinctively the plants that helped.

In their book on the ethnobotany of Britain and Ireland, *Medicinal Plants in Folk Tradition*, Allen and Hatfield wrote of a body of evidence which shows 'that the folk medical tradition was impressively wide in its botanical reach and equally impressive in the range of ailments it treated'. They also noted that 'roughly half the world's pharmaceutical products in use today are plant-derived ... There is still much to be learned from native plant medicines.'

Herbal cures still exist in Ireland, but most of the people who have them make just one cure using a few wild plants. They make the cure as it was told to them and they are generally not aware of how or why it works. Only 20 per cent of the cures I investigated involved the use of herbs and many of these herbal cures also included a blessing or a prayer. Faith cures are much more common; their proliferation is most likely filling the gap which has been created by the gradual loss of our herbal lore over the past 170 years, since the Famine.

At the beginning of the twenty-first century in Ireland we are almost totally reliant on drug companies and pharmacists, doctors and hospitals to meet our medical needs. We seem to have lost the large body of healing knowledge that our ancestors built up over generations, which helped to keep them alive and healthy. In 2019 I was teaching a class of six-year-olds in a large town in the north-west. Having read them a story of a caterpillar who developed an upset tummy, I asked the children how their parents could help them if they had a similar problem. They proceeded to name a number of pharmaceutical products, and to look at me blankly when I suggested warm milk and honey!

## Herbalists

Dr Henry Purdon visited Belfast vegetable market in August of 1895 and came across a herbalist's stall there selling a broad selection of healing plants. He commented 'many persons are to be found who prefer the advice and treatment of the herbalist to that of the registered and qualified medical man'. Traditional herbalists are becoming very rare in Ireland. I searched extensively, but was only able to locate a few people who fit into this category; healers who have a comprehensive knowledge of herbs (passed down through the generations) and who use their skill to cure a variety of ailments. Wise women in previous centuries were suppressed and persecuted, and this no doubt is one of the reasons why the herbal healing tradition has struggled to survive. Professor Gearóid Ó Crualaoich has written that in Ireland, 'Many accounts exist of the tension between wise/healing women and Christian clergymen who regarded ... in some cases ... the wise healers as witches ... somewhat deranged, prone to pagan superstition ... a danger to her community.'

However, I did interview one interesting elderly woman who was a traditional herbalist and healer. She lived on a hill overlooking a pretty cove on the west Cork coastline. From her home she ran a tiny, eclectic museum overflowing with unusual artefacts, stones and bones. In her healing work, which she had been doing for more than sixty years, she used two approaches, herbs and her hands. 'I am very proud to be amongst the list of healers. I was born with the gift ... you can't learn it,' she said. When she was a child, she used to fix injured hens, maybe a broken wing, and gradually she realised that not everyone could do this.

Her mother taught her about plants, how to identify them and their healing uses; 'she took us into the fields, and she pointed out all the plants and we listened'. When making her preparations she felt it was more effective to use fresh, wild herbs. 'I don't dry the herbs and store them for the winter because they lose their medicinal qualities.' She gathered the plants she needed in the fields surrounding her cottage, preferably in the morning and in dry weather. There were different herbs available in each season and one could always be found for the required cure, even in wintertime when the land appeared barren.

People came to see her and following a discussion of their problem, she made up a herbal bottle for them. 'It's important to see them, to look at their eyes and their skin ... their hair ... when you are in pain you look older.' She simmered the selected herbs in water, stirred frequently, and sealed the resulting liquid in a sterilised bottle. In addition, she tried to find the source of the 'hurt' and to work on that area of their body with her hands. 'I use the pressure of thumbs ... energies come from my hand and the area gets red [and hot].' She understood that her herbal cures were beneficial to many conditions, including skin problems, boils, ulcers, asthma, the kidneys, blood pressure and heart disorders.

She wanted to pass on her knowledge, preferably within the family; 'my nieces are interested and they know a lot'. She was completely immersed in her herbs and healing work, and found great reward in it. 'It's not a burden ... you are a better person if you have helped someone ... you feel so happy when you see them coming back looking different, looking younger.' I believe this woman was unique in Ireland, as she was one of the few to carry on the tradition of healing using herbs, a contemporary *bean feasa*.

I also visited a traditional herbalist who ran a successful herbal medicine practice in a large market town not far from Dublin city. His family had been herbalists for five generations and he hoped to pass the skill to his children. I was unable to speak to this man in person, but I was given a tour of his modern clinic by a younger colleague. They primarily used Irish herbs, ones that were grown on their farm locally or better still collected in the wild. Some plants they travelled to find, as with horsetail (for hardening of the arteries) which was gathered on the Shannon flood plain in Leitrim. The business worked hard to be as self-sufficient as possible; therefore, they saved the seed from their plants to sow the following year and used spring water from their own wells to make the herbal remedies. He used the same healing herbs that his forefathers trusted: nettles, comfrey, hawthorn, meadowsweet and ox-eye daisies.

## Skin Cancer

Dr Patrick Logan wrote in 1972 that, 'The treatment of skin cancer is one of the specialities of folk medicine and one where for long the folk curer enjoyed considerable success.' This is no longer a common cure in Ireland. It appears to have died out in the north-west, so I travelled a long distance to speak to someone who is still making it. The man I interviewed was a middle-aged farmer in the south-east. His uncle gave him this popular herbal cure; it had been in his family for over one hundred years, and he believed that it was originally bought by a great-aunt for £100 from a Mr Green.

He said that the skin cancer could be on any part of the body; often it was on the arms and legs. His cure was a plaster (paste) which he made from plants gathered locally. 'The herbs, I pick them along the beach and I pick more at the back of the sheds, they're everywhere.' He collected these plants once a year, every summer, 'May or June … it's enough to keep going … I wouldn't use a lot of herbs … [it is a] very small plaster.' He used four different herbs and he kept their identity secret. Once the herbs were gathered, he had to 'dry them … grind them, and mix them together' using specific quantities of each plant. There were no prayers involved in this cure; it was totally herbal.

Those in need of his help were welcome at his home Monday to Friday between 6 p.m. and 8 p.m. He could make his cure any day and at any time, but due to his farming and family commitments these hours suited him best. When people visited him initially, he always advised them to seek a second opinion, to see a doctor. However, if they wanted to go ahead with the cure, he started it immediately. He was honest with those who requested his cure. 'I tell them straight ... can we sort this or can we not.' He could not assist people who had already had medical intervention. 'I have to get at it first, not after a doctor's biopsy', and he also said that if the problem had 'gone too severe ... I wouldn't touch it'.

Following an examination of the skin cancer, if he felt he could help the person, he put a small herbal paste onto it; '[it's] like mustard ... put it on ... put some gauze over it and the yoke of an egg ... that wets it ... that binds it ... that will stay on pretty well'. He asked them to keep the plaster dry. He had been making this cure for twelve years and had grown more confident about it: 'I'd know exactly now how much herbs to put on ... you don't want to leave any marks on people ... so you go as gently as you can.'

A second visit would take place ten days later. He would then remove the herbal paste; 'just take off the plaster, see that it has done what it was supposed to do'. He then would put a regular (band-aid) plaster over the area, and tell them to 'go home and poultice it'. This part of the cure was challenging as it involved time and dedication. A fresh poultice needed to be applied to the affected skin, 'every three hours ... [for] six to eight weeks'. The poultice was made by putting a piece of white yeast bread (batch bread) into a cup with hot water. The water was drained off, and the warm, damp bread placed on the skin and held in place with a plaster. He said that it usually took 'six poultices ... a day' and that one should be left on at night too. He thought that 'the yeast helps to clean it out ... that it'll heal'.

When these weeks had passed, the person would return for a third and final visit and to check that 'it's all gone'. He told me that at this stage the cancer growth would normally come away from the body, including the roots, which can be painful. This man believed his cure to be very successful; occasionally he would make it a second time, for 'the real bad ones'. He said that often 'a small mark is left behind', but people did not mind this as they were happy to be cured. He could pass on his cure to a woman or a man, not necessarily a blood relative, but he was most likely to keep it in the family and give it to one or all of his children.

There was also a woman in her seventies in the south-east, in a neighbouring county, who had a similar cure, but hers did not involve the use of poultices. She inherited the cure from her mother twenty years earlier; 'it's in the family for many generations, my mother, my grandmother and her mother'. It had been passed down along the female line, but she felt it could equally be made by a male member of the family. 'I suppose the women have more time and they're in the house.' She hoped her daughter would carry on the tradition.

People rang her to enquire about the cure and to discuss their concern. If she thought she might be able to help, she invited them to her house. Most of the people who came to her had decided to try the cure before modern medicine. After the first visit, 'If there's anything I know that I can't cure, I will send them to a doctor.'

Many of the cancers she treated were on the face, so the herbal paste she applied was 'very discreet'. Egg white and a piece of gauze were used to stick the paste to the skin and to keep it in place. This herbal plaster was left on the skin for at least three weeks; 'it remains on for three weeks to six weeks ... and around that time it should fall off and it [the cancer] will be gone completely'. The person then returned to her. 'I'll have a look at it, it may need to be dressed for a while ... there's a sort of hole ... that has to heal.' She told me of an old man, with cancer on his chin, whom she had made the cure for three months previously. His skin had healed up very well. 'It was lovely, as clean as a whistle!' she recalled.

She helped on average ten people per year, some locals and many strangers, from Tipperary, Carlow, Kilkenny, Dublin and farther afield. She had huge faith in her cure and believed its success rate to be '100 per cent, absolutely ... a cancer has roots ... my cure will kill from the root ... it won't spread.' She felt that the herbs caused the cure to take place, but she prayed for its success as well. This was her personal adaptation of the cure. 'I would also be praying ... every time I think about them' and some people remained on her 'prayer list a long time'.

She was taught by her mother how to make the cure and the wild herbs required were available in her area. But she still used plants that her mother dried and left for the cure, and she thought these herbs remained potent. She expressed concern about the possible contamination of plants due to current farming practices, by the use of fertilisers and weed killers; 'you want to be careful where ... [you are] picking up the herbs'. This woman had great respect for and love of the natural environment within which she lived, a beautiful river valley. She believed that herbal cures are a gentler approach to healing and she said that 'out there [in nature] all the cures are, for everything'.

## Shingles

I spoke to a young woman (in her late twenties) who lived in a sleepy village in north Leitrim. She was the mother of three small children and had a cure for shingles. Her cure was a mixture of thirteen plants found locally: 'It's ... just herbs that you pick, that are growing in the fields and ditches ... it won't do anybody any harm ... it's just all natural.' Over the summer months she would gather the necessary plants. 'Gathering the herbs, it can take weeks ... and sometimes it's not easy ... one year ... I was heavily pregnant in the summer; it was a killer making it.'

Once she had a sufficient quantity of herbs, she would make the cure. It took almost three days to prepare a large batch of the cure. It could be quite strong smelling, so she made it on a gas ring in an outside shed. She put the plants into a large pot and added unsalted butter. 'Simmer it for about thirteen hours to get all the green, all the herbs ... then you have to strain it.' Once strained, she poured the warm liquid into numerous small, plastic tubs, where it cooled and hardened to resemble a green 'soap'; it was then stored in a fridge.

People were directed to rub the cure on their shingles twice daily, morning and night, until it was all used up. If the rash disappeared but the pain remained, they should keep applying the cure. The cure came with a sheet of 'silk proof paper' (thin, light plastic), which was placed over the treated shingles to prevent clothes sticking to the herbal 'butter'. The affected area had to be kept clean and dry, and the salve was not to be washed off. She also advised people to take vitamin B complex following the cure, as they were often in poor general health and sleeping badly.

This cure was completely herbal and unlike most traditional Irish cures there were no prayers connected to it. However, the last line of the directions which accompanied the cure stated, 'Hoping, please God, you have relief from pain.' This woman gave the same advice as those who had the cure before her. Twenty years earlier I had interviewed her neighbour who, at that time, made the cure. I was pleased to see that this cure had survived and that it was still very popular.

Not far away there was an eighty-year-old man with a comparable cure for shingles. He had a second herbal cure for 'The Rose' (erysipelas) and he made an ointment to cure ringworm too. He was given the three cures by an old woman (not a relation) from a nearby village, two decades before I interviewed him. To make the shingles cure he had to gather wild plants in the surrounding fields, 'nine different herbs ... some of the herbs that I had always treated as a menace about the place ... I treat them with respect now,' he said.

This was his most popular cure and he had people looking for it every month, including 'three or four within the past week'. Over the years this cure had travelled to every part of Ireland and it had been brought to the USA. When I asked him how people knew of his cure, he smiled and replied using the Irish phrase, '*dúirt bean liom go ndúirt bean léi!*' which translates as, 'a woman told me that a woman told her!'

He was determined to pass on his cures, and had already shown one of his sons how to make the cures; if any of his other children were interested, he planned to tell them as well. He wanted to see the traditional cures continuing and believed that it would be 'a loss to the area' if they were to die out. He said, 'that's all they had some years back and they seemed to do very well ... They must have found out what's in these herbs ... and it has prevailed down through the years.'

## Jaundice

I met a south Sligo farmer (in his fifties) who had a cure for jaundice. It was a herbal cure which he made with the assistance of his wife. They welcomed me into their home for a cup of tea and a chat. When I was a child, I had taken this cure; at that time, it was being made by his uncle who lived in my local village. I recall that it had an unpleasant taste and I found it hard to drink. 'It's still not nice to take because it's bitter ... I think it's the herb,' he said.

He made the cure using convolvulus (bindweed), which grew abundantly around his farmhouse. In summertime he would pick its leaves, in wintertime he would dig up its roots. 'It takes longer ... when you have to start digging for the roots; it's easy enough when you can go out and pull the stuff green.' The cure took about an hour to make and in addition to the herb, he used one litre of milk and four half pint bottles of beer. He charged no money for it, but when people came to collect their freshly prepared cure, they were asked to bring these two ingredients with them, so that he would have them in stock for the next cure.

He boiled the milk and beer together, washed the convolvulus, chopped it finely and added it to the boiled liquid. After a thorough stir, the liquid was strained through muslin and the juice squeezed out. To finish the cure, he added a secret ingredient. The greenish liquid was left to cool, then bottled; there was generally less than two litres remaining. He instructed people to take a teacup of this herbal drink in the morning before breakfast until it was all gone, about seven days later. He advised them to avoid full fat milk while taking the cure; 'we were told as it was handed on not to let people drink full milk with it ... it would sicken your stomach'.

In the years just before I spoke to him, he had made his cure infrequently, but was willing to do so if asked and to 'hope it would help'. He believed it to be quite effective; 'it has down the years cured a lot of people'. He felt that if the problem was jaundice and nothing more serious, it should have started to improve after 'three or four mornings ... the eyes would clear'. Allen and Hatfield documented the traditional use of bindweed in Fermanagh as a remedy for kidney problems. They also wrote that hedge bindweed was used in Northamptonshire (the English midlands), and that '"the poor people" were still boiling the roots in ale as a purge as late as the 1830s'.

In an earlier chapter I mentioned a woman with two cures, strain and jaundice. She was a grandmother and farmer, and she kept a little homestead on the slopes of Sliabh an Iarainn (mountain of iron) in south Leitrim. Her jaundice cure involved prayers and herbs. Unusually, the number eight was central to her cure. She had to gather eight plants (all of the same type) and touch the person with the plants on eight different parts of their body. 'You ring me ... I'd have to go out and get the herbs ... eight of those herbs ... out of the bog ... on me own land.' In winter it could be harder to get the herb, and if the ground was frozen, she asked her son to help. She showed me the small plant that she collected; she called it simply a herb and was not aware of its name.

The sick person would then come to her house, and she started the cure by saying five Our Fathers and five Hail Marys in honour of

St Benedict (St Benedict thistle was used to treat jaundice). She stood in front of the person while she was saying these prayers and put her hands on their shoulders. Then she touched eight parts of their body, their skin, using a different plant each time. As she was touching them, she made the sign of the cross using the herb. 'You have to rub them on the forehead ... on the breast ... the back, between the two shoulders ... the forehead again ... the two hands [palms] ... the soles of your two feet.' This procedure took 'about five minutes' and afterwards she burned the eight herbs. To complete the cure, she would see the person twice more and repeat this ritual, on Mondays and Thursdays only.

She had had this cure for twenty-five years and was given it by her mother-in-law, via her late husband. It had to be passed from woman to man, to woman, and she planned to give it to her son. She thought that many people combined the doctor and the cure; they 'go to the doctor first ... when they hear that they have the jaundice, then ... they go looking for a cure'. This woman would not accept money for either of her cures: 'I don't ever take money for cures ... that's the tradition ... years and years ago ... when the cures started ... people that time had no money to give anyone.' She lived a quiet life, and enjoyed meeting and talking to those who came for her cures. 'I often give them a cup of tea,' she said, before they have to give up milk as part of the cure.

I interviewed a retired businessman in a large town in the north-west; for many years he ran a well-respected fishing and hunting shop. Over the decades his family had made a popular cure for jaundice, which people requested and collected from the shop. It was a herbal bottle (based on milk), and the sick person was directed to keep it in the fridge and to drink it over three days, each morning fasting. The cure had to be taken, 'in the name of the Father, the Son, and the Holy Spirit'. Avoidance of alcohol and salty meat was recommended while taking the cure. It was best if people started the cure as soon as they felt unwell, and he believed they were normally fully better within two weeks.

The belief in the cure was so strong in his town that some people thought it was enough just to ask for the cure and to receive it, but that there was no need to take it. 'They then came to me ... and I made it for them, they could take it [home] ... and empty it down the sink!' He described this practice as 'throwing it out', and had found it very frustrating as a lot of time and effort went into making the cure. He also said that, 'You got very little feedback, it was like the ten lepers. One in ten might come back and give you a present.' In her folklore collection *Visions and Beliefs in the West of Ireland* (1920), Lady Gregory recorded a jaundice cure which was to pick worms from the earth of a freshly dug grave 'boil them down in a sup of new milk and let it get cold; and believe me, that will cure the sickness'.

## Kidney Stones and Gallstones

There was a man in his thirties who worked as a carpenter and school bus driver in rural Sligo. People were often surprised when they realised that he was young; 'they associate cures with older people,' he said. His well-known herbal cure was for gallstones, stone in the kidney, and jaundice. All three conditions used the same cure, and about 70 per cent of the cures he made were for gallstones, 30 per cent for kidney stones, and it was rarely used for jaundice.

To make the cure, he went into the fields surrounding his house and gathered or dug up the required plants. In the winter, 'the ground is frozen and it's harder to work'. In the summer, 'when I come home in the evening, I can go out and make one ... It's a pleasure to go out.' The number nine was closely associated with this cure. He had to collect the herbs in groups of nine. He then brought the plants into his kitchen, washed them, and simmered them in water for nine minutes. Next, he strained the herbal liquid, allowed it to cool and bottled it. The process took around one hour and he could prepare up to three cures together. The cure was divided into nine small bottles and one of these had to be taken every morning fasting for nine days; before the cure was drunk a blessing was said. The bottles were numbered one to nine and the person drank number one on the first morning, number two on the second morning, and so on.

Another aspect of the tradition was that the bottles were supposed to be small, empty whiskey ones. He referred to a baby Powers measure and even if the nine bottles varied in size, he always used this measure to fill them. He asked each person who came for the cure to bring nine small bottles with them; these he kept and used for the next cure. 'It's just the way it was handed on to me and I … follow what was written out by me mother … and it works.' Instructions came with this cure which included keeping it refrigerated, starting to use it as soon as possible, and not eating eggs or smoking while taking it.

I spoke to a man who was a farmer and retired bus driver in south Leitrim. He had a gallstone cure too and occasionally people used it for kidney complaints. His was a totally herbal cure which could be made whenever it was requested. He felt that most people had been diagnosed with gallstones before they came to him and that they were trying to avoid surgery. He said that it was not an easy cure to take, but 'it seems it's able to dissolve them'.

Unlike other herbal cures that I researched, this man did not go out into the local lanes and fields to collect the plants, rather he bought them pre-prepared from an international supplier. He was not exactly sure what the herbs were, but it was the same mixture that his father used twenty years before. He brought the herbs to the boil, simmered them for a while and then left the liquid to cool down. The cure came in a large bottle, and people were instructed to drink half a (whiskey) glass of it first thing in the morning and last thing at night, until it was all used up. It took five or six days to finish and sometimes people came back for a second bottle. He believed that the continued popularity of his cure indicated that it was successful.

## Vertigo

I interviewed a middle-aged trade union official from south Sligo, who was enthusiastic about the traditional cures; he was planning to write a book to record them, in memory of his mother. 'My mother had huge interest in cures ... in herbalism' and she had encouraged him as a child to respect them. He had three cures, for burns, colic (which has already been discussed) and vertigo. He was shown how to make the vertigo cure by his mother; 'my mother brought this plant home from England'. He grew the same scrambling plant at his home, and to make the cure he cut off part of it, 'a twig' and instructed people to 'wear it around [their] neck' until they felt better, which was 'generally three or four days'. He gave them enough of the plant to do this and advised them to 'sew it into a scarf'.

He was clear in his belief that he could not take money for his cures and that to do so would negate them. If people insisted on giving money, he suggested they donate it to a charity of their choice. Some people brought him gifts; they 'believe they must give you something' and usually it was food. He fondly remembered a woman who returned unexpectedly after he had cured her child of colic, with a bottle of wine and a leg of lamb. People 'from all walks of life' got his cures and they also contacted him if they were looking for one: 'I have a little book ... I keep the names of the different people who have cures ... and I have that book of knowledge in my head.'

He believed that the source of the healing in his cures was God. 'It's not me ... I just happen to be a conduit ... there's a greater force ... which is God for most of us Christians ... for somebody else it would be some other power, but it's a greater power.' He thought that if someone was given a cure, 'they give it to you for a reason, and if you have it, you have a responsibility to use it'. He told me that having these cures has had a very positive effect on his life.

## Erysipelas

Deep in the hills of north Leitrim a grandmother lived in a little cottage with a lovely garden. She had two cures, a faith one for a sprain and a herbal one for 'The Rose' (erysipelas). The latter is a bacterial skin infection which causes large, raised inflamed areas, often on the face, but it can be on the arms or legs too. She used one common (secret) herb to make her cure, 'the top of it … it's a weed,' she said. She gathered the plants close to her home; 'they have to be in season … [that is] from spring to [when] the frost kills them'.

In her kitchen, she crushed the plants into small pieces, then mixed them with unsalted butter. Using her hands, she formed this green herbal butter into 'nine wee balls' and as she was doing this, she said some prayers; 'naturally you think of them [the sick person]'. She instructed those receiving the cure to rub three butter balls per day on the ailment, for three days in a row. They were not to cover the area with bandages or clothing and had to avoid washing it. The cure could be started any day of the week and the butter balls rubbed on individually throughout the day. In the past this cure had been popular, but recently there had been little demand for it.

Erysipelas used to be known as St Anthony's Fire. Beatrice Maloney documented (in the 1970s) a poultice made from boiled chickweed as a traditional Cavan cure for the condition. One hundred years ago Dr Blake had noted the use of bog mould 'an excellent antiseptic' as a cure for erysipelas. I was intrigued to learn that during the First World War (1914–18) large quantities of sphagnum moss had been collected from bogs across Ireland, primarily by women volunteers. The University College Dublin Archive records that, 'Irish Bogs contain an abundance of a particular type of moss known as sphagnum which has antiseptic and absorbent qualities.' The moss had been sewn into cloth dressings for wounds and then sent to the battle hospitals of France, Belgium and beyond, to provide life-saving and healing treatment to hundreds of thousands of young men.

## Piles

There was a retired woman in west Sligo who had a herbal cure for piles. Her mother-in-law had made it before her. 'I knew to see her making it ... when she died ... people came and said did I know about it', so she restarted the cure. When the cure was requested, she would go into her garden and dig up the roots of a particular plant. She could identify this herb, but was not sure of its name, 'just a small, green leaf on it and in springtime there's a little, yellow flower'. Once indoors, she washed the roots to remove any clay, then simmered them with a small quantity of petroleum jelly 'for a good while ... so that they soften ... whatever juices are in it ... they come out'. Next, she removed the roots from this liquid and poured what remained into containers, where it cooled to an ointment consistency. She advised people to apply it as needed.

This woman told me that the roots of the plant, 'they're the shape of what piles would be', so I think the herb in question is most likely lesser celandine, also known as pilewort. She had noticed over the years that the herb had become difficult to source as lawns have become more cultivated, and that it was easier to find in older gardens and wild spaces. She got good feedback on her cure; however, she acknowledged that, 'maybe you don't always hear from the people that it doesn't work for'. She thought that in her area quite a few cures had survived but she said too that much of our traditional healing knowledge has been lost; 'they say there was a cure for everything'.

Allen and Hatfield recalled that in the Highlands of Scotland lesser celandine roots were applied to small breast lumps. Also, in Cornwall and Antrim this plant was used as a cure for piles, and 'a decoction of the roots, applied with very hot compresses or as a mild ointment, has earned medical respect as an excellent remedy for haemorrhoids.' Phil Cronin recorded an ointment made from pilewort as a treatment for piles in Mayo: 'The leaves and flowers were mixed with unsalted butter and applied.'

## Burns

I met a woman in east Leitrim who made a burn cure; she was in her forties, a homemaker and mother of seven children. The cure was a mixture of herbs gathered locally and combined with butter. 'Mammy gave me the recipe ... they're very common things, out through the hedges ... handfuls of everything.' Once she had the required herbs, the names of which she kept secret, she put them in a pot with butter: 'You just boil them until you think ... all the good is gone out of them.' She then strained the liquid into a large glass jar.

The cure was made in the summertime when the herbs were plentiful and stored in the fridge. She had some to hand the day I called by; it was a green/yellow, solid salve, with some sediment at the bottom of the jar. She said that the 'cream' will soften at room temperature and that the heat of the burn will melt it. When she gave the cure to someone, they were told to apply it 'a few times a day ... to put it on and keep it on', until they felt the burn was fully healed. She recommended that they place a bandage over it.

All who arrived at her house to collect the cure were welcomed; 'they come in and sit down, and have a mug of tea'. She believed her cure to be effective; 'it kills the pain very quickly and it leaves no scar'. This cure was looked for more often when her parents had it; there were no longer many callers for the cure, but she still kept it ready in case it was needed.

## Whitlow

I spoke to a middle-aged, articulate woman who lived on a farm in a north Cavan mountain valley. She had a herbal cure for 'whittle', which she said was an infection of the fingers, usually of the joint close to the nail. This problem can be very painful, with the joint becoming red and swollen, and in severe cases requiring amputation. Medically the condition is known as whitlow and it is often caused by a prick or a small cut which becomes infected.

She made the cure with a commonly available herb. She mixed the herb with a secret ingredient; 'it has to be made into a paste for to stay on'. Prayers were said as she prepared the cure and these were kept secret too. People tended to phone her to enquire about the cure and to order it; she made it fresh for each person. The cure was applied once daily for three days and as it was being put on, they said a blessing. Non-religious people could omit this prayer and she felt that it would still work. The person was instructed to refrigerate the cure, not to wash the infected finger, and to keep the paste covered with a bandage.

In general, the cure worked quickly; 'they say once they put it on the pain ... eases'. Occasionally, the infection 'can be harder to shift' and people returned for a second cure. She felt that a belief in the cure contributed to its success. Children and adults had received her cure, and though the numbers she helped were low, people had travelled quite a distance to get it (from Dublin and Meath). Cronin wrote that both a white bread poultice and plantain (in Irish, *slánlus*, health herb) were traditional remedies for whitlow, for the latter 'the leaves being washed, soaked in hot water and wrapped around the finger'.

## Comfrey

Comfrey has a long-established reputation for reducing swelling, healing damaged tissue and repairing broken bones. It has been an important plant in the traditional herbal medicine of many European countries, known popularly as knitbone or boneset, and in Ireland as *lus na gcnámh mbriste* (herb of the broken bone). Nicholas Culpeper, the famous seventeenth-century English astrologer-physician, wrote of how the 'great comfrey ... for outward wounds or sores ... is special good for ruptures and broken bones ... so powerful to consolidate and knit together'. Allen and Hatfield highlighted that comfrey 'is rich in allantoin, which promotes healing in connective tissues through the proliferation of new cells'.

Dr Logan recorded that a poultice of comfrey roots was a standard method to treat sprains and bruising, and that in Kerry it was also used for boils. Phil Cronin documented that a 'paste made from comfrey roots was sometimes applied to breakages ... This was spread on a strip of gauze and applied to the injury ... The properties of the root ensured a successful knitting together.' In the recent past comfrey was utilised by some country people as an animal fodder, in particular for pigs. Today, many gardeners use it as an organic fertiliser and its flowers are loved by the bees.

There was a grandmother in a small town in County Sligo who made a herbal gel from comfrey leaves. She had found it to be helpful to arthritis, general aches and pains, leg ulcers, and for dry skin, rashes and psoriasis. She did not inherit this cure; as a child, seventy years earlier in south Leitrim, she remembered her father having huge belief in the healing abilities of comfrey. He had used it for pains and strains, and had cured a horse with a sore hoof. He made a paste from comfrey leaves, 'put it on the hoof ... bandaged it up ... in two or three days the whole thing had healed'. Many years later she came upon a solitary comfrey plant in a garden centre, 'that is surely meant for me ... I brought it home and planted it.'

When people came to her for the cure, she would give them some of it to rub on their ailment, a few times each day and for a short period of time. In the case of leg ulcers, the gel was not to be put on broken skin, rather it could be rubbed carefully around the open sore and 'as it heals ... bring it closer and closer in'. The oily leaves that she discarded when the gel was made were a poultice for painful joints, especially for the knees and elbows. She had been making this cure for five years and had given it to 'about two hundred people ... from different parts of Ireland'. She was happy to help others and wanted nothing in return. 'I've met some lovely people ... they've all been very grateful ... it's been a great experience.'

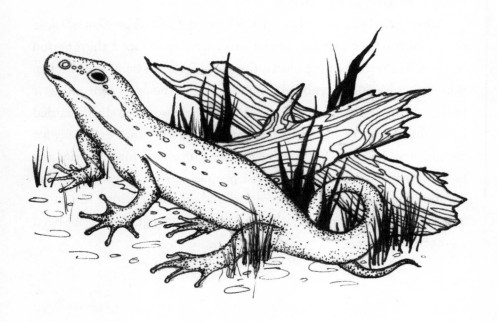

*To acquire the cure of the burn, you must lick a mankeeper (the smooth newt). They live in damp, dark places, such as at old wells and under log piles. Then, you can lick a burn and heal it.*

# CHAPTER 8

# INDEPENDENT CURES

# Burns, Eczema, Shingles, Whooping Cough and Warts

I HAVE CLASSIFIED A SMALL number of the cures I investigated as 'independent' cures. By this I mean cures that cannot easily be placed into the faith or herbal categories. However, many of these cures incorporate a blessing or a prayer and the person making the cure may feel that the source of the healing is God; therefore, they have a faith component.

## Burn and Lick

If you want to possess the cure of the burn, you must lick a mankeeper. This was the traditional name given to a smooth newt; a small amphibian, about 9 cm long, with four splayed legs, a long, sturdy tail, mottled brown in colouring and paler underneath (sometimes orange).

It is the only Irish newt species. These elusive little creatures are usually found in damp, dark places, such as at old wells, in weedy ponds or under timber piles.

Once you have licked the newt you can then lick a burn and heal it. If we get burnt, for example on the hand, we may instinctively lick it, so this is possibly why the cure is made by licking. This cure was recorded in County Louth in the 1930s and is part of The Schools' Collection; the belief was that if a person caught a 'man-creeper … and licks his belly three times and swallows the spittle each time he will be able to cure any burns' (NFCS 664: 85). Peter Kavanagh, a native of Monaghan, wrote in the 1950s that a newt was called a 'man-eater; he is feared because he may jump into your mouth, go down to your stomach and live there eating the food'. Mankeeper is probably a corruption of man-eater. Dr Logan has written that the licking of a burn was a 'very primitive form of treatment … the explanation is that the tongue of the licker has acquired a poison from the animal and this poison is able to overcome and drive out the poison that is in the burn'.

I met with an elderly woman who lived in the south Sligo countryside and had a popular cure for burns. She acquired this cure in childhood when she licked a mankeeper that she came across in the bog. Her mother had told her about this old belief. When people received a burn, they came to her as quickly as possible and she licked it. She had noticed that even if the burn covered a large area, she always had enough saliva. The pain disappeared once she licked the burn and any blister subsided. If the burn was severe, she advised the person to get medical attention.

She has never picked up an infection while performing her cure, although now and then it had been difficult to do. Over the years she had helped hundreds of people, family, work colleagues and many strangers. She felt that her cure was always successful and she had great faith in cures generally; 'the cure is different to the doctor ... If you get cured with a cure, you're cured.'

I also spoke to a man in his late forties with the same cure; he was a farmer, an electrician and a community activist. As a boy, his father had encouraged him to lick a mankeeper. To make his cure he explained, 'all I do is lick the wound ... lick around the wound ... and I get the person that is burnt to bless themselves three times and I bless myself once'. He said that his cure would remove the pain from the burn and that no scar would be left, unless the burn was very deep. He recalled an occasion when he had used his cure to assist a local man whose hand had been burned by molten metal; 'he was in dreadful pain ... so I took off the dressing and I licked it, and he blessed himself and I blessed myself'. Two days later he met the man again and he was much improved, the pain was gone. This man believes that 'with cures no money should change hands ... because it is a gift ... people say it is a gift from God'.

There was a man with cures for colic and vertigo, whom I have already written about. Both he and his wife had the cure of the burn; they had licked a newt. Sometimes they made it jointly, in particular if the affected area was large. Interestingly, he had adapted this cure as he was told by his sister, who had been making it for many years; 'you don't actually have to lick [the burn] ... you can lick your own thumb and make the sign of the cross with your thumb [on the burn], and that will work'. But he stressed that all of the burnt skin must be touched with the thumb (or licked) and that any part which was overlooked would not be cured. He said the old explanation for this cure was that the mankeeper had developed a 'belly of flame'. He elaborated by saying that 'they [the newts] live in the bog and bogs were traditionally burned in Ireland ... the belly can't get burned ... they can slide over flames ... That's what my mother would have said.'

In the long, hot summer of 2018 I was informed by a hairdresser that she had recently got the burn cure and had found it to be helpful, to have taken away the pain and accelerated the healing process. She had got badly sunburned on her back, chest and arms. A customer noticed her distress, and said that her husband had the cure and could help. So, this middle-aged countryman duly arrived at the hair salon (in a County Sligo town), licked the sunburn and repeated the cure the following day. 'I don't know which one of us was more embarrassed!' she said.

## Burn Ointment

I interviewed a married couple who both made cures, for a burn and a 'mote in the eye' (as mentioned earlier). They lived on an elevated, rocky plain in south-east Sligo, the site of a great mythological battle. I was welcomed into their house, supplied with lots of tea and told of their cures. The woman's burn cure was an ointment made from equal quantities of unsalted butter and sheep suet; she melted them together. The mixture was left to cool, then a third (secret) ingredient was added, something that was bought in a pharmacy. 'There's prayers I have to say as well when I'm making the cure', which remained secret also. When the liquid was still warm it was poured into glass jars; 'I give out small portions ... very little does [cures].'

She showed me some of the cure; it was a cream-coloured salve of thick consistency. People were directed to rub on the ointment, 'about three times ... morning and evening, and the next morning again'. Thirty-three years previously her mother-in-law had given her this cure. They believed it was more than one hundred years old and had been passed down through the female line of the family; they felt it could possibly be given to a man, but most likely she would pass it to her daughter-in-law who lived nearby.

Close to a small town in north Roscommon there was a retired man who had a similar cure for burns, using mutton. He made it every few months and stored it in the fridge. There were no prayers attached to this cure. Those who got the cure were instructed to melt it a little and to dab it on the burn, 'if the skin isn't broken'. If it was a 'bad burn', he recommended they soak a bandage in the greasy ointment and then wrap it around the damaged skin. The cure had to be left on the burn for nine days. This man believed that his cure worked well and that the pain would go from the burn as soon as it was applied. In past years this had been a popular cure, but more recently people had seldom asked for it. He had inherited the cure from his father, who was given it by a neighbouring woman, and he thought 'it could be going back generations'.

Patrick Logan described a common treatment for a burn in Cavan/ Leitrim as having been a preparation of one part of beeswax to three parts of mutton fat. He explained that 'mutton fat has a high melting point, as has the bees wax. When the plaster is applied ... it becomes soft and forms a smooth airtight cover for the burn, so preventing secondary infection unless the dressing is removed ... the burn will heal quickly.' The plaster was put on as soon as possible following the burn. He noted that in some instances the dressing was to be left undisturbed for nine days.

Lady Gregory, in the early 1900s, wrote of a Galway man, Conolly, whom she was told 'knew every herb that grew in the earth'. He had many cures including one for the burn: 'He boiled down herbs with a bit of lard, and after that was rubbed on three times, he was well.' Lady Wilde, in the late 1800s, documented a burn cure: 'Take sheep's suet and the rind of the elder-tree, boil both together, and the ointment will cure a burn without leaving a mark.'

## Eczema and Ringworm Ointments

I spoke to a woman in her seventies who lived on the outskirts of a large midlands town; she had cures for eczema, bleeding and sprain.

How she made her eczema cure was kept secret, but she said that it was an ointment created using ingredients that she bought. When someone phoned her to order it, she established the severity of the condition and the amount of salve they would need. She did not have to see the individual with the problem, and the freshly made cure could either be collected or posted to them. The ointment had to be applied sparingly to the eczema twice a day, morning and afternoon, until it was all gone; the affected skin could not be washed during this time. She felt that after one week the condition, which was often chronic, would have started to improve; the eczema would begin to flake off. The salve she made was well-known; every month many people came for it, especially teenagers. They travelled from different regions in Ireland for her cure, but particularly from Donegal, Roscommon and Sligo.

Cures for ringworm are generally associated with the seventh daughter/son tradition; however, I did come across one which was an ointment. This cure was made by an elderly man whose herbal cure for shingles I have already explored. Exactly what he used to make the salve was a secret, but he did tell me that he had to mix four ingredients together, 'some that you can buy in the chemist'. He kept the cure in the fridge until it was required. Locals collected the cure and he posted it to those living farther away. He thought it was an effective cure for ringworm, adding that some people had complained that it stung, 'but still it got rid of it'.

## Shingles and Blood

In rural Monaghan there was a young grandmother with a shingles cure. She normally had a telephone conversation with anyone looking for the cure before they came for it, 'because they have to bring the rooster'. As part of the cure, she took blood from a rooster's comb. She did not supply the rooster; those who wanted the cure had to find one and bring it to her. And she would not use the same rooster more than once a year as she liked to give him a rest: 'the rooster has done the cure along with me'. Occasionally, down through the years she said that roosters had escaped and flown off into the countryside, never to be seen again!

This cure was made over three consecutive days, and the rooster had to be taken away and brought back each day. She cut a different part of the comb each visit and collected the blood. 'I just have a little scissors and cup, and I hold it [the comb] real tight, it doesn't do any harm to them … I have to get a good bit of blood.' She would then dip her finger in the blood and rub it all over the shingles. She would make the sign of the cross with the blood three times on the area of skin that looked the worst, silently saying a blessing each time. On the second visit she only rubbed the blood on the shingles, and on day three both parts of the ritual (the blood and the blessing) were performed. People were told not to look at or touch the shingles and not to wash off the blood for the duration of the cure. After the third day, 'you can see the shingles start to go away and gradually the pain goes with it'.

When a sick person came to her initially, she would ask them questions about their shingles and the possible cause. She believed there was a reason why they got shingles, a psychological dimension to the physical illness. People could be run down, depressed, worried, 'deep down there's a reason'. This woman had been making the cure for thirty years and was given it by her mother. It had originally come from north Donegal where her grand-uncle lived; 'My mother got it from her uncle … from Tory Island … it's very, very old.' She hoped to pass it on to one of her children, probably her daughter. Her belief in the cure was strong and she said that even if the person receiving it was sceptical, 'it will still work because I have the belief … I know in my heart that when I do the cure for them, that the pain will go … I know that I can cure.'

I also talked with a farmer and builder in south Sligo who had a shingles cure which utilised blood, his own blood. In order to make the cure he had to prick his finger and draw blood, and then mix the blood with a small quantity of butter. He tended to take blood from the middle finger of his left hand; 'you have to get a fair amount out,' he said, as he liked to see 'a red stain in the butter'. It could be a slow process to get enough blood, so often he sat down, relaxed, and watched TV as he was doing it. He wrapped the cure in tin foil and left it in the fridge until it was collected. He instructed those with shingles to 'rub it on the affected areas … and hope for the best' and to do this for a few days.

This man believed that his cure 'relieves the pain … and it starts to dry up' and that with time the problem would disappear. He was eligible to make this cure from birth because his mother had the same surname as his father before they married, but he did not commence doing so until he became a teenager. He had been making it for five decades and over those years had helped many people, 'two or three some nights'. As with most cures there were busy and quiet periods, but the demand never stopped. He said that they 'always bring you something, a gift, and some of them would give you money'. A lot of those that requested his cure were strangers, from the surrounding counties, and it had been taken to England and the USA.

Mac Coitir wrote that in the past in Ireland people with particular surnames were believed to have special healing powers: 'the blood of a Cahill could cure shingles, while the blood of a Keogh could cure ringworm'. He recalled that Keogh had been an eighteenth-century Anglo-Irish herbalist. Logan alluded to an old belief which was that members of the Keogh family could heal St Anthony's Fire (erysipelas); they had to rub their blood (Keogh's blood) on the infected skin. He commented that, 'The use of blood as a method of treating disease is very ancient.' Dr Logan also noted that shingles was treated using 'fasting spit' (the morning spit, before breakfast); whoever was making the cure rubbed their spit on the blisters and then made the sign of the cross over the shingles with a blessed wedding ring. He understood that, 'Fasting spit has an important place in the history of medicine and it is used for many conditions.'

## Whooping Cough and Ferrets

I met a man in his mid-forties who lived in the heart of an old port town in the north-west. He had a well-known cure for whooping cough which he was able to make because he kept ferrets. The ferrets were pets and sometimes used for hunting rabbits. Those who wanted the cure brought one litre of milk to him. He then gave his ferrets some of this milk to drink for three days. Each day, whatever milk the ferrets did not drink, he collected, strained and bottled. This was known as the ferret's 'leavings' and it was the cure.

The milk had to be drunk by the person with the whooping cough, usually a child, for three days in a row. He felt that even a small amount of the ferret's 'leavings' was sufficient to cure. 'Give them a teaspoon of it,' he suggested. Many parents put it in the baby's bottle at night when the cough could be worse. If people were local, he gave them the ferret's 'leavings' each day, but if they lived a distance away, he stored it in the fridge and they picked it up on the third day. Often, he would come home from work to find milk and a note on his doorstep.

When I interviewed this man, he had seven ferrets in cages at the back of his house. He cared for them well and handled them regularly. He brought one into the living room for me to hold as we were chatting! The milk for the cure was separate to their daily diet. The ferrets were divided between a few cages and he gave different animals the milk each day. He left the milk for the cure with them for less than ten minutes; 'if you leave it in too long with them, they'll topple it over'.

He did not know how his cure worked, but he remembered the old people saying years ago that the cure was 'in the ferret's tongue'. In my conversation with Sligo GP Patrick Heraughty in 1986, he had suggested that possibly the saliva of the ferret contained an anti-spasmodic. During my research for this book, I was teaching in a little country school in south Sligo and while there I was shown copies of former pupils' contributions to The Schools' Collection. The same cure for whooping cough (they called it chin cough), using the food a ferret left behind, had been recorded by the children collecting folklore in 1938. Dr Blake, lecturing in 1917, referred to this cure and its popularity in his part of County Louth, 'for ferret's milk in this instance does not mean the mammary secretions of the sporting beastie, but the milk that has been given to it as food, and out of which it has drunk'.

## Warts — Sell and Forget

I spoke to a ninety-year-old man with a wart cure; he was a former cattle dealer and lived in a market town in north Leitrim. I enjoyed listening to his stories about the cure, which he had had for more than sixty years. To get rid of warts, he first rubbed each of them, then asked the person would they sell them to him. People of course readily agreed to this offer. He gave the person a large safety pin in exchange for their warts and told them to put it in a place where it would never be found or interfered with: 'It's very important ... hide that pin ... put it in a wall ... or bury it.' He asked them to say a prayer of their choosing when they went home, and he said a few prayers for them and for the success of the cure. In 1896 Dr Purdon had written of a wart cure from County Down which utilised nine pins that had to be 'thrown away or dropped into some holy well or stone cavity'.

There was a woman (in her forties) in a small town in south Sligo and she too had a popular cure for warts. She touched each wart with her hand, by making the sign of the cross on it. It was crucial that she touched all of the warts; if she missed any, they would remain. After she had done this, 'you have to look them in the eye and you say, your warts will be gone in three weeks'. If it was a child, she got down to their level to impart this significant message. She said that people were rarely embarrassed, no matter where the warts were; 'their mind is focused on this ... that they have to get it'. This woman could also cure a foot verruca (a wart) in the same way, but she was asked to do this infrequently.

She thought it was best if the person forgot about their warts having received the cure. 'What people have told me is that generally they don't notice them going ... they kind of forget about them, and the next thing they wake up and look, and they are gone!' Similarly, a seventh daughter, who cured warts and ringworm, told me that it was very important (to the success of the cure) for people to try to forget about their warts after their third visit to her.

In Donegal, a man who had a bleeding cure felt that the traditional cures had remained strong in his area and he knew of people who had them. He talked of an old man with a wart cure; 'he has to count' them. A lad went to this man with over thirty warts on his hands and 'by the time he got home all the warts were black' and gone within a week. Logan commented on the proliferation of folk remedies for warts, which he said were 'simple, cheap and quite effective'.

## The Shilly Shaw

On the rocky coastline of north Sligo, I had a conversation with a middle-aged farmer. He had an unusual cure which he called the 'shilly shaw'. He made it for adults who had been extremely hoarse for a long period, weeks or even months. 'It's an Irish name for severe hoarseness ... a rare enough sort of a problem,' he said. I consulted an Irish language (Gaeilge) scholar, who felt that the term shilly shaw was most likely an anglicisation of the Irish phrase *sine siáin*, which translates as 'the tit of the inside throat'. This is the uvula, and the dictionary describes it as the 'small fleshy finger-like flap of tissue that hangs in the back of the throat ... an extension of the soft palate'. Inflammation of the uvula can cause discomfort.

This man was very secretive about how he made his cure. He believed 'you tell someone how it's done when you're passing on the cure' and not before. But he did say that the 'cure is part herbal, part religious and part faith' and that it took about one hour to make. Touch was a component of the cure. 'I have to lay me hands on them.' This cure was made over three days, 'between sun up and sun down, and never on a Sunday'. The visits occurred every second day, 'Monday, Wednesday and a Friday would be ideal.' He felt that by day two, an improvement should have occurred in the condition.

The cure had been in his family for eight generations and in excess of two hundred years; he was given it by his grandfather. It had been passed down along the male line, but he said that 'could have been just the thinking of the time'. He said he would consider giving the cure to a woman in his family (the next generation) in due course. This problem was also known as the 'fallen' or 'dropped' palate, and Phil Cronin documented a cure for it in Mayo which involved pulling 'certain hairs on the crown of the head' and placing a hard-boiled egg on the head, held in place by a scarf 'to be worn for a number of days and the patient was advised to talk as little as possible'.

# CHAPTER 9

# Cures for Animals
# and Bone-setting

IDDY EARLY, THE FAMOUS NINETEENTH-CENTURY Clare healer, was remembered for curing lots of animals. Edmund Lenihan, author of *In Search of Biddy Early*, unearthed stories of her helping farm animals and their owners: 'The loss of a pig or calf could mean the difference between payment and non-payment of rent ... The death of a working-horse could spell destitution ... many of the queries brought to Biddy's door related to the health and welfare of such animals ... vets and medicines ... were more than half a century in the future.'

Allen and Hatfield wrote that 'more than a hundred different herbs are on record as having been used in Britain or Ireland to treat ailments of animals', and that many of the 'remedies tried and tested on them' would have been used to treat humans as well. Up until the middle of the twentieth century Irish country people continued to rely considerably on traditional cures (that they or their neighbours possessed) to heal their domestic animals. It was not until the 1970s that people began to

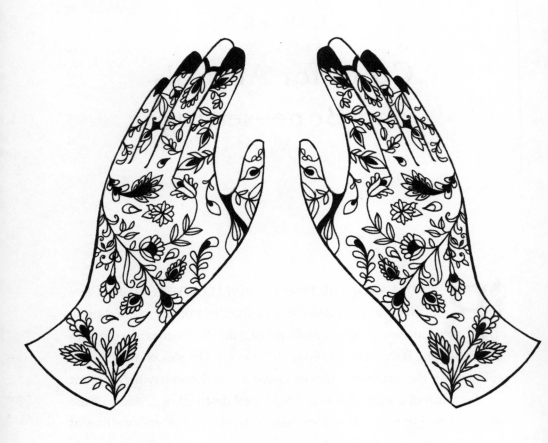

For the calving paralysis cure, the young woman went to the cow that was 'down', usually in a cattle shed. She circled the animal, touching her continuously (the back and legs) as she prayed.

significantly use the services of vets; this coincided with our joining of the EU and a gradual increase in the prosperity of rural Ireland.

My research at the start of the twenty-first century found that many of the cures (including herbal knowledge) for animals have been lost. Today most farmers rely almost totally on veterinary surgeons and pharmaceutical products to maintain the health of their livestock. Twenty-five per cent of those I interviewed healed animals, but their cures are used to help humans too; only three of the ninety-three people I spoke to made cures exclusively for animals. The art of bone-setting is also struggling to survive in modern Ireland. However, the cures that continue to be utilised are fascinating and the following accounts are based on my fieldwork.

## Bleeding

I interviewed a woman with a cure for bleeding who was a grandmother, homemaker and farmer. She regularly made her cure for cows that were calving, and in the past for cattle that had been de-horned. It was a prayer cure and she needed no information about the person, the animal or the problem. People generally telephoned her to request the cure and 'I say the prayer ... straight away.' It took only a few minutes to make, but she had to focus on the words. 'I would keep repeating it a few times, in case I didn't say it sincere enough ... in case it didn't get through the first time.' Often, she stood alone at her kitchen window looking out onto the fields as she recited it. Her prayer recalled Jesus and the River Jordan, and the final line commanded the blood to stop 'in the name of God'; she always put emphasis on the final word 'stop'.

In the late 1960s, having returned from London to live and farm in south Leitrim with her husband, she became aware of the cure. They had a new-born calf that would not stop bleeding. 'My brother-in-law ... said to go and see a man in town ... he had that cure.' Her husband went to this man, 'he read the prayer' and to their amazement the bleeding stopped. This man had made the cure for her mother as well 'whenever she had serious nosebleeds'. He gave the prayer to her mother and she passed it to her daughter. She did not see herself as having the cure, rather as having the prayer to make the cure; 'it's just a prayer and it's the same for anybody to say it'. She was willing to tell the prayer to others, 'if someone really wants it'. This woman was modest about the success of her cure, but she was aware that it had worked numerous times.

A farmer and fisherman, in his early fifties, lived on the edge of a hillside town in south Donegal. He too had a bleeding cure which he made for people and animals. Over the past fifteen years he had been asked to stop every sort of bleed. For animals, that included cuts, internal bleeding, complications with dehorning and castration, and 'redwater'. For people, it had been accidents, nosebleeds, brain haemorrhages, bleeding ulcers, vaginal bleeding, knife cuts and gunshot wounds. He thought that many people did not go to their vet or doctor when the bleeding started; instead, they phoned him for the cure.

If he was making the cure for an animal, he required five pieces of information: the owner's name, the sex, age and breed of the animal, and the type of bleed. If it was for a person, he had to know their name, sex and age and the nature of the bleed. Once he had these details he made the cure, which was a special prayer, and it took 'less than a minute to say'. He had memorised this 'unusual' prayer and kept it secret. He said the prayer silently or aloud, depending on where he was. 'Most people ring me ... I could be at sea in the boat ... or having a drink' in the pub. Whatever the location, he gave the cure priority and made it immediately. He said the prayer only once, but if the person had severe bleeding, 'I would say it ... several times.' People were told to phone again if they need the cure repeated.

This was a popular cure, especially within his community. 'I would say ... yearly, fifty or sixty.' He kept a 'book' in his house where his wife and children wrote down requests for the cure if he was not at home. He took nothing in return for his cure. 'I was told you don't accept anything for it ... I feel that if you start taking stuff for it, the cure won't work.' This man, the youngest of nine children, inherited the cure from his mother; 'she wanted to pass it on before she died ... She asked me if I would take it.' He had to give the cure to a woman, but when I spoke to him he still had to choose his successor; 'I have to hand it on to a female ... and hope for the best that they'll do it ... if I pass it on tomorrow then it's over, it's done with me.'

He felt that belief in the cure, by those receiving it, was important; 'if people believe in it, the power of healing is huge'. However, he personally held some doubts about his cure. 'I think I believe in it; I can't be 100 per cent ... maybe it would have healed up anyway?' He described his cure as 'coming from faith' but he was not religious. 'I don't pray to God ... except when I make the cure.' 'The way I look at life is I try and do nobody any harm ... if I thought I'd help them ... I'd cured them ... put somebody at ease ... you feel good in yourself that you are trying to help ... I just do my best.'

In an earlier chapter I discussed a cattle dealer who had an extremely popular cure for haemorrhaging. An organiser of the mart in a small Leitrim town told me a story concerning this man and his cure. One day at the mart a horse cut her hoof and the vet could not stop the bleeding. Twine was tied tightly around her leg and it had little effect; 'it was gushing'. So, he rang the cattle dealer and asked him to make the cure. A few minutes after when he came back to the mare, he found that the bleed had ceased, and she was subsequently sold.

I know a vet who in the early 1990s encountered the cure for bleeding while practising in Kilkenny. He was called to a farm where a large bullock was bleeding heavily from a cut on the face. He worked on the animal for a long time, cauterising and suturing, but was unable to halt the flow of blood. Finally, the farmer's wife (a nurse) intervened and asked would he mind if she telephoned for the cure. He had no objection and the woman left the yard to make the call. By the time she returned, five minutes later, the bleeding had stopped. The bullock was given a transfusion because it had lost so much blood and survived.

Professor Michael Doherty conducted research among Irish veterinarians in the late 1990s. He examined the vets' experiences of folk custom and belief, particularly with regard to the treatment of cattle diseases. His findings showed that there was still widespread use of the bleeding cure to help with any type of haemorrhaging or babesiosis (redwater, blood in the urine). For example, a Tyrone vet recalled that, 'On getting a call to a haemorrhage case usually after calving, the farmer would ring a local woman immediately who was said to have the cure for bleeding. She required some description of the cow, colour, breed, location, etc. By the time the vet arrived at the farm the bleeding was invariably under control.' The bleeding prayer reported by a vet from County Westmeath in this study is almost identical to one I recorded in Leitrim. And the wording for a prayer to stop redwater, documented by a south Monaghan vet, is very similar to the bleeding cure prayer I came across in that area, with the exception that the redwater version was followed by nine Hail Marys.

## Orf

I met a sheep farmer whose home was on a wild mountainside in east Leitrim. She had a cure which was for orf, foot rot (severe lameness) and angleberries (papillomatosis, warty growths on the skin); she was best known for curing orf. This is a viral disease that affects sheep and lambs; 'it's very nasty … blisters come on their mouths … on their udders' and the lambs are unable to suckle and can die. It is contagious and can spread quickly within a flock. People may contract orf from sheep and occasionally she made the cure for a person. 'It could be anywhere ... on your hands ... like a round ring ... [it is] itchy and very sore.'

Farmers usually phoned and asked her to make the cure for their sheep. In order to do so she needed some information: 'the [farmer's] name and the number of sheep'. She had to know the name of the farmer who owned the sheep and the name of anybody else who worked with the sheep, often a son or daughter. She also wanted to know the exact number of sheep with orf, because if a farmer had seventeen sheep sick, but told her that it was fifteen and she only made the cure for fifteen, then only fifteen sheep would be cured.

This woman was unable to tell me how she made the cure; that knowledge was reserved for whoever she decided to pass it to. 'I can't say what is involved ... I might do some harm to it [the cure].' However, she did tell me that she had to make it out in the fields during daylight hours, on Thursdays and Mondays only, and that the procedure 'takes at least ten minutes'. Her cure was a combination of a herb she gathered and prayers she said, though she believed ultimately it was a faith cure: 'the prayer I say with it must be what cures'.

She said that she made her cure more for the farmer and the family than for the sheep; she felt that the cure works through the people to their animals. The time it took for the animal to recover varied; 'some ... it's gone in two or three days ... more of them, it might go on for maybe a week, or three weeks'. This cure was popular, particularly in the spring; 'in springtime I could have anything up to twenty to do' and to make twenty cures in one day could take her over three hours. 'I love sheep ... and no matter how busy I am, I have to do it for them ... you feel like you're compelled to do it.'

She was given her cure 'from a neighbouring man across the hill'. The old man wrote down the cure and sent it to her. 'I do always think of him when I go out to make it ... I wouldn't like to let him down.' She was not sure why he chose her, but 'I think the reason [was] ... because he said I was a great woman with the sheep ... I was able to take good care of them.' This cure must be passed on to a man, and she knew that she would have to make her choice wisely, as she would only give it to someone who would 'be very dedicated ... likes animals and likes sheep'.

## Calving Paralysis

There was a woman in north Cavan who was a mother and farmer. Her cure was for calving paralysis; 'it's when a cow gives birth ... and they remain down ... their back two legs get paralysed'. She said it was a common problem and that sometimes the cow could be 'down' for a week before the farmer phoned her. Her late father had given her the cure thirteen years previously. He was very ill and unable to make the cure for her brother's cow, 'so I just says to Daddy ... to give him peace of mind ... give me the cure, and I'll go out and do it'. He had a tattered piece of paper in his glasses case with the special prayer written on it. 'He handed it to me ... and he told me how to do it.'

To make the cure she had to travel to where the animal was and just one visit was necessary. She would bless herself to commence the cure; next she circled the cow slowly and repeatedly, rubbing her and praying; 'I keep in ... contact with the animal all the time ... saying the prayers.' Using both her hands she touched the cow, on her four legs and along her back, and 'all the time you're praying'. She said the cure prayer and then recited the Creed three times. This set of prayers was repeated twice more and a blessing finished the ritual. It took up to twenty minutes to complete the cure, and she would ask the farmer to be quiet while she was doing it so that she could concentrate on the prayers.

She advised them to tie the cow's hind legs close together to ensure that they did not spread when she tried to stand up, and that they had plenty of straw under her. She believed the cure to be quite successful and that the cow should stand 'within three to four days'. 'Some I would get an inspiration ... I think it [the cow] will make it ... some ... I don't think they will.' Her cure was 'a seasonal thing', calves are born from spring to the end of summer and she made it on average once every two weeks during that period. This cure involved a lot of travelling to farms around Counties Cavan, Leitrim, Fermanagh and Longford. 'I don't mind ... it's just to get time to go for it ... I'm always rushing!' She had to juggle her commitments to her children, home and work.

She told me that the cattle may be nervous or she might be alone with them, but 'I'm not afraid because I was born and raised on a farm.' This woman was kind to the animals and generous to the farmers. She accepted no money for her cure, not even for petrol. Now and then 'they'll come out with a bag of goodies to the kids in the car'. She had a lot of respect for and belief in the traditional cures; that was the way she was reared. 'Daddy was always a great man for the cure.' She thought people must have faith in the cures for them to work, including her own. This cure had to be passed from a woman to a man, to a woman; she said that when the time came, she would give it to her son. 'I'd like to keep it within our family.'

Vet Michael Doherty's folklore research describes the use of garlic to help a 'downer cow'. To cure this problem a few farmers in Ulster still insert a clove of garlic under the cow's skin, near the top of her tail. A County Antrim vet documented that 'a cow down for several weeks after calving last spring, 1999, the farmer asked a man from the Glens to look at her, he incised the tail and inserted garlic and she was up the next day!' It was also reported that a similar method of treatment was used in the past in County Dublin, with the addition of a red flannel wrapped around the wound for seven days.

My grandmother Helena (born in 1893 in north Galway, who lived to one hundred) was a great believer in a red flannel to protect the chest and inner organs, and to keep oneself healthy. Fleetwood wrote in 1951 of the influence of John of Gaddesden's medical books on Irish healing practice; he was a celebrated fourteenth-century English physician. This doctor claimed to have used a red cloth to cure smallpox: 'Then take a scarlet or red cloth, and put it about the pox; as I did to the King of England's son when this disease seized him and I permitted only red things to be about his bed, by which I cured him.'

In 1963 Waterford woman Dervla Murphy cycled alone from Ireland to India. Having caught her breath, she volunteered to work in an orphanage for Tibetan refugees in the Himalayan foothills. While reading her account of this challenging experience, I came upon her description of the children wearing around their necks 'a picture of His Holiness [the Dalai Lama] and a piece of red cloth blessed by a High Lama and guaranteed to protect them from evil'.

Patrick Logan referred to the traditional use of red cloth for healing, writing that red 'is the colour which is believed to resist the power of evil spirits ... red cloth [was] tied on the tails of cattle to protect them ... and the use of red flannel in folk medicine is also an example of this very ancient belief in the power of red things'. He remembered that when he was growing up in the 1920s in south Leitrim (close to north Cavan) and a heifer calved 'there was a special elaborate ritual carried out to make sure she would do well'. He described how the hair on her udder was singed with a blessed candle, and then the lighted candle was 'passed across her back, under her belly, and then backwards between her hind legs'. He concluded that, 'All this is clearly a combination of pre-christian and christian rituals.'

## Foot Rot

I spoke to a woman in her late sixties who lived in Leitrim; she was a homemaker and sheep farmer. Her cures were for pain in the back and sprain, and for foot rot. She explained that foot rot is an infection which can be exceedingly painful and cause lameness; it affects cattle, sheep, horses and donkeys. The cure involved prayers and dandelions. She was clear that the dandelions must be of the 'single root' variety; 'if I got a wrong herb, it wouldn't cure'.

When the cure was requested, she cut ten dandelions in her garden using 'a black-handled knife'. As she was cutting each one, she would say three prayers, a special, secret cure prayer, an Our Father and a Hail Mary. She brought the tenth dandelion into her house and later gave it to the farmer. They would be instructed to rub it on the infected hoof in a downward motion, 'towards the ground' and to bury the dandelion afterwards in the earth. This part of the cure was most likely based on the concept of transference, where the problem is believed to be transferred to the ground, and as the plant decays and disappears, so too does the infection.

She had adapted her cure to accommodate farmers who lived far away or who had cattle that were unused to human contact. In such instances, she would cut the dandelions and say the required prayers. Usually, she placed the tenth flower on the windowsill for a few days, 'leave it wither away ... I do bury it myself in a soft place ... in the garden.' Also, she made her cure any day of the week if 'the animal was bad', whereas it used only to be made on Mondays and Thursdays.

Her father-in-law gave her the cure and she had to pass it on to a man, maybe to one of her sons or her son-in-law. The cures were part of her family's history and they had remained in the same location, which had been significant for their survival. People who received the cures in the past had returned to the old house looking for them, and they had found them next door with this welcoming and caring woman.

She told me that a traditional cure for foot rot was to walk behind the limping animal with a spade and at the exact spot where the swollen hoof was placed, dig up and turn over the sod of clay; this act was repeated three times, and the third and final turned sod was thrown away. In 1997 Doherty photographed a Meath farmer performing this ritual of 'turning the sod'. He described how 'the animal with foul [severe lameness] is watched, the imprint made by the lame foot is identified, a circle is cut round this with a penknife and then the inner core of this circle cut out'. This sod of earth was then taken to the perimeter of the field and thrown out, while a prayer was said. He wrote that this practice is likely to be hundreds of years old, and 'may represent a symbolic transference of the disease "in the sod", taking it out of the animal and away from the field. This is a theme that is common to traditional or primitive medicine throughout the world.'

## Pink Eye

Another Leitrim woman I interviewed was a grandmother in her seventies. She lived in the south of the county, near a market town where she ran a pub for many years. She had five cures, four of which were for animals, pink eye (keratoconjunctivitis), calving paralysis, foot rot and sprain. She made her sprain cure for people too, and one for a stye in the eye. Her most popular cure was for pink eye, a contagious eye infection in sheep and cattle; 'the eye is festered ... it waters a lot ... Once one gets it, others get it.' All five cures involved prayers and they were made in a similar way.

Most people telephoned her, described the problem and asked her to make the cure. She would then go to a quiet place, generally her bedroom, to say the prayers. She said a different prayer, 'a special prayer', for each cure. 'I say the prayer three times and the Creed, and then the three prayers again.' She repeated these seven prayers twice more, at different times, to complete the cure. 'I usually do it three times ... I'd make it this evening ... tomorrow morning and ... tomorrow evening again.' She kept the special prayers secret and believed this was an important element of the cure. 'I wouldn't like to betray it [the cure].'

She said that she would only tell the prayers to the person she decided to give her cures to.

This woman had been making these cures for more than thirty years. People were continually requesting them, especially the ones for pink eye and sprain. Those who phoned her were mostly strangers, from all over Ireland and occasionally from the USA. She got little reward for her cures as she did not accept money and was rarely given a gift in thanks. 'I never hear from them again ... until the next time they have something wrong.' She said, 'I just like to help people ... that's what we were put on this earth for ... if you can't do that for people, what the hell good are you!'

## Bone-setting

In times past the tradition of bone-setting was strong in Ireland. However, in recent decades it has weakened dramatically. The dictionary defines a bonesetter as 'a person who sets broken or dislocated bones, especially one who has no formal medical qualifications'. They may not have studied their subject in college, but these healers had considerable knowledge and skill, usually handed down within their family. They also learnt through prolonged observation and practice, and for many there was a strong intuitive component to their healing work.

Dr Logan thought highly of the traditional bonesetters. He wrote that:

> One of the great skills of the bone-setter was his ability to pull the fragments apart without causing much pain to the patient ... it is then necessary to replace them so as to restore the original line of the bone. This is often a matter of great skill and only long experience can enable the bone-setter to know when he has done it properly.

Folklore collector Phil Cronin recalled that the late Anne Cronin, from Crossmolina, north Mayo, was a well-respected bonesetter. She had inherited the skill from her grandmother and had passed it on to her husband. She was able to treat dislocated joints in the shoulder, hip and finger: 'she carefully studied the injury and slipped it back into place by skilful manipulation. In the case of breakages, she made a plaster of flour and beaten egg whites which she wound around the broken limb after setting it in place'. Apparently this family tradition of bone-setting ended in 1993, with the sudden death of Anne's son.

In the 1970s Anthony Buckley conducted research into unofficial healing in Northern Ireland, and he concluded that 'both herbalists and bone setters are extremely rare'. My fieldwork in the early decades of the twenty-first century concurred with his view; these two very old forms of folk medicine appear to be dying out in Ireland. With regard to bonesetters, I found it difficult to locate ones who were alive and well and using their skill. A handful of bonesetters still exist in Ireland, but their numbers are declining with each decade. Having said this, I did interview a few people who were part of the tradition, including one man in the south-east who had a great reputation nationally as a bonesetter.

He was an arable farmer with a passion for racehorses, and had been bone-setting for almost fifty years. He said that this healing work had been 'in the family for generations', possibly four hundred years. His uncle, grandfather and great-grandfather all practised it. Following the death of his uncle he was asked to help a little girl with a dislocated wrist. 'I had no notion of starting ... I was very doubtful.' But the child's father persuaded him to help, believing he was able to carry on the family tradition: 'Go and do it, and don't let down the name; you're the only one left now.' So, he obliged, and 'I felt something there in the wrist ... gave it a little twist, it clicked back in ... that was the beginning.'

Since then, he had been helping people, initially on a small scale, but gaining experience, confidence and popularity with time. 'I was seven or eight years doing it and I wouldn't look at a back, afraid I'd do some harm.' Later he primarily helped damaged backs; 'slipped discs are the biggest problem'. He advised people with this problem 'to be extremely careful the first three or four weeks' after visiting him and to take care of their back for six months, 'then you'd be as good as ever'. He held a 'clinic' at his house most afternoons and normally people visited him once. Some came from England, and he said, 'If the pain is bad enough, you'll travel; distance is no object.'

He told me that bone-setting 'means replacing dislocations, backs, ankles, knees, shoulders … you can splint a break' using light timber, 'a dislocation you just bandage it up'. He had helped many animals, including horses, cows, dogs and cats. This man had no medical training and believed that the art of bone-setting could not be taught; 'as far as I'm concerned you don't learn it … you just feel [the problem] … and push it back into place … that's how it works'. His sister was a bonesetter too, though she did not use her skill regularly. He hoped a few of his children would continue the tradition. He also thought that there were not many bonesetters left; 'there was one nearly in ever county … two or three in some counties … [they are] disappearing fast'.

His bone-setting work was respected the length and breadth of Ireland. In general, he felt it to be 'very successful … if it wasn't working … they wouldn't be coming'. He believed his skill was 'a gift from God … through me … It's purely a gift from God, nothing else.' Even though he was getting older, he was still healthy and hard-working; 'I might get physically tired, but I stay going … It's very satisfying to think I have helped so many people … that's what keeps you going.'

I spoke as well to an elderly man in a large town in the north-west whose healing work was part of the bone-setting tradition. He had no medical education and did not inherit his skill, yet he had worked successfully for five decades with local football teams treating sports injuries, pains and strains. 'It's hard to explain, but I have a feeling ... something that's in my hands ... I can feel what no one else can feel ... you have a gift.' He seemed to understand intuitively what was wrong with the person and how best to treat them.

He had been interested in healing since he was a child; 'if there was a bird injured, I'd try and help ... I often put wee splints on a cat ... I was always meant to do it ... you have to have the *grá* [love] for it.' He developed his skill and knowledge as a young man, learning about anatomy, movement and injury while working as a butcher. For years he had given help and advice to local athletes, such as go to the beach and wade in the sea; fifteen minutes in the water followed by ten minutes walking on the sand, and repeat; 'salt water will take away swelling in two or three days'. Massage of the damaged area was a core part of his treatment, using his own oil preparations of olive, wintergreen, and chilli oils, and sometimes a little *poitín* (moonshine).

He had a good relationship with the doctors and orthopaedic consultants in his town, who occasionally recommended people to him. However, he encouraged everyone, if at all possible, to 'keep away from the knife [surgery]'. This man was no longer able to work and his skill had not been passed on within his family. But he still thought of all those he had helped; 'I'm happy with what I done ... I loved doing it ... I loved helping people.'

In a multicultural market town in south Galway there was a friendly butcher who was also a bonesetter. In 2018 I talked to him in the little shop he owned there. He said that he had started bone-setting more than twenty years previously and that for him the skill was not hereditary, rather he unintentionally and gradually began to do it. He was now well-known for his healing work and dedicated one day of the week exclusively to it. He told me that if I returned the following day at 8 a.m. there would be a queue of vehicles down the street, those looking for help from him. In the morning he worked on people, whatever aches, pains and concerns they presented with. The afternoon was for injured animals, often horses, and greyhounds seemed to be his speciality.

He had not had medical training (though he was a skilled butcher), but he knew intuitively, with his hands and mind, what the problem was, if and how he could help. Interestingly, he always spoke of 'We' – we know this, we do that – and he believed that he was not alone when he carried out his bone-setting work. I asked him did he mean God and he replied that he was not sure, that he was not a religious man, and he felt it could be explained more as a positive acknowledgement of 'Right' or 'Good'.

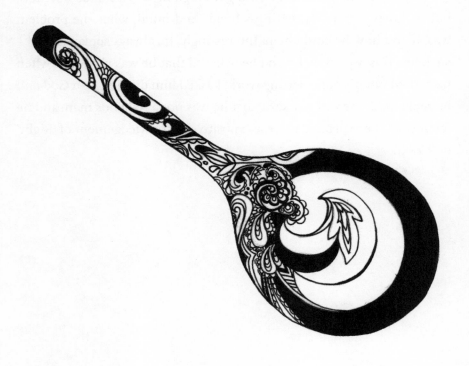

*To cure mumps, she put a rope halter around the sick person's neck and led them to a mountain stream. She gave them stream water to drink, on a spoon, and they both said prayers.*

# CHAPTER 10

# Acquisition of Cures

FROM MY RESEARCH I FOUND that there are primarily two ways of getting a cure in Ireland: by having the cure passed to you or by acquiring it because you meet certain criteria. Of the 119 cures I investigated approximately 75 per cent fell into the first category; they had been passed down through the generations, often within families, and many from woman to man, to woman. Some cures are also given to people by their neighbours and friends, and occasionally by strangers. Almost 25 per cent of the cures I examined had been acquired by the person because of the existence of specific circumstances, in particular at the time of their birth. Within this category there were four distinct subdivisions; seventh daughter/son (which I have already discussed), posthumous child, breech birth, and a woman and man with the same surname marrying.

These are the general 'rules' for obtaining a cure, but variations exist from place to place and from person to person. However, most of those I interviewed believed that the way in which they had got their cure was the correct one. Buckley, following his fieldwork in Ulster, concluded that, 'To use a cure, one must be entitled to use it, and one must therefore have acquired the cure according to clearly defined rules.' I was interested to read his findings and to see that the categories of acquisition he identified in the 1970s were very similar to the ones I came across thirty years later.

## Passed-on Cures
### Woman to Man, to Woman

The majority of traditional cures in Ireland can be passed on. Of the cures that I explored which were of this type, nearly 30 per cent of them had to change sex each time they were given to someone new; so, if a woman had a cure, she could only pass it to a man and he in turn must give it to a woman. Having said this, the length of time someone holds on to a cure can be brief, once the gender stipulation is fulfilled each time the cure changes hands. A good example of this would be one woman's plans for her head fever cure, a cure that 'has to be passed on from a man to a woman'. Her father had brought the cure with him when he moved from the countryside to the town where she lived. It had been briefly given to her mother, then her late brother, and she had been making it for over two decades. She intended to pass the cure to her daughter, but she said it would first have to go for a short while to her son-in-law and thereby adhere to the tradition of its acquisition.

## Family Cures

Many cures are handed on within families; the figure was almost 50 per cent of all the passed-on cures in the research that I conducted. Sometimes the reason a cure remains within a family is because that is part of the tradition of the cure. But it is more likely that people just want to keep their cure within their family; they view it as part of their family's heritage and inheritance. If they can only pass the cure to one person, they usually like to give it to someone who is close to them, often the next generation, their child or a favourite niece/nephew.

The requirement to change gender every time the cure is given to somebody new is also common in this situation, as in the case of the man who had a faith cure for blood pressure and heart fever. This cure had been in his family since the 1960s and he had been making it for more than twenty years: 'It was my mother passed it down to me.' He planned to give it to his daughter or granddaughter. 'It has to be passed from a woman to a man ... to a woman ... I will pass it on ... to a female member of the family.'

Other family cures I investigated included a herbal one for gout. The woman (in her early eighties) who made it was living in a small County Sligo town, but her cure originally came from east Donegal, the place where her husband grew up; he had been given it by his sister. After her husband died people came looking for it, so 'I kept it up ... I knew how to make it.' She told me that she intended to pass on her cure to someone in the family, and while I was writing this book that is what she did; she gave the cure to her son in west Sligo.

## Non-Family Cures, from Neighbours, Friends and Strangers

A cure can be given to somebody by a person they know but are not related to, generally a friend or neighbour. Less frequently people get cures from strangers. Twenty-five per cent of the passed-on cures that I researched came under this non-family cure heading. Again, within this grouping the condition often exists that the cure is passed from woman to man, to woman. I met a man who received his heart and headache cures from a person who was not his relation. She was an elderly local woman with whom he was friendly and she had no children. He was worried that the cures might not survive so he asked her for them. 'I thought to myself, it's a pity to let those cures die out ... I just said to her this day ... will you pass on that cure to me? ... she did.' Since then (fifteen years), he had been happily making these popular cures.

In Tyrone there was a man who was given heart fever and sprain cures by his late wife. The heart cure originally came from the other side of the border, from Donegal. His wife had gone to get this cure for her mother and while there she was asked would she take it. The woman who had the cure said that her children were all living abroad and that she was 'tired doing these cures, and me husband is not well ... and nobody wants it'. So, his wife graciously accepted.

## Acquired Cures
### Posthumous Child

In Ireland there is a traditional belief that if a child is born after their father's death they will have the cure of 'foul mouth', which is thrush (candidiasis, an oral fungal infection). To make the cure the person must breathe three times into the mouth of the sick individual, often a baby, and they usually bless themselves or say a prayer. It is a short procedure, normally repeated for three days, consecutive ones, or Mondays and Thursdays.

Dr Logan noted that thrush was a relatively new infection to Ireland, exacerbated by the rise in bottle-feeding and the use of antibiotics; however, the 'curing of a disease by breathing on the sufferer is very old in medicine'. Therefore, this cure can be taken as an example of how old healing practices are sometimes applied to new ailments. It suggests that the traditional cures are not static, rather that they change and adapt over time to meet people's needs. Dr Blake, addressing a gathering in Dundalk in the early 1900s, stated that there was a simple cure for thrush 'so common in young children, especially artificially reared infants ... It is only necessary for a child that has never seen his father (i.e. a posthumous son) to breathe upon and spit fasting spittle into the patient's mouth.'

I interviewed a farmer in south Sligo who had been making a thrush cure for more than sixty years. I knew of this man by reputation as he had healed my twin niece and nephew when they were babies (2001). He acquired the cure of 'foul mouth' because he was a posthumous child. He started making his cure when he was very small; 'the lady next door ... she had a sore mouth, and I was so young the only thing she could ask me for was a kiss and I was in me mother's arms'. He was a thoughtful man and did not like to keep people waiting, so when they phoned about the cure, he recommended that they come to him as soon as they could. 'Six to seven in the evening is always a sure time of getting me here ... it's milking time ... a lot of the cures be administered in the dairy!'

He made the cure by breathing three times in the child's mouth and saying a blessing. With the first blow into the infant's open mouth, he started to bless himself and he said, 'In the name of the Father'. As he breathed the second time he said, 'and of the Son'. The third and final blow into the mouth concluded the blessing, 'and of the Holy Ghost, Amen'. He was never told a particular way to make his cure; rather, he settled upon this simple method himself.

This man's cure was made over three days, Thursdays and Mondays only, 'between the hours of sunrise and sunset'. Now and then he made the cure after sunset if that suited people better. And he preferred that they visit him three times, but if the child was only brought to him once or twice, he respected this decision and felt that the cure must have already worked. 'Some will tell you that there is nearly an instant response; maybe others won't have it as fast.' He recalled a toddler who arrived with a very sore mouth, unable to eat or drink; just after the cure, to her mother's amazement, she asked for an ice cream.

There was a soft-spoken woman living in a large town in the north-west and she too had a cure for thrush. She made it in a comparable way; she breathed three times into the person's mouth and then said three Hail Marys. This short ritual was repeated three days in a row, and she warned that 'you can't skip the days … if they miss a day, you have to start all over again'. For fifty years plus she had been helping people with this cure. As a younger woman she made it fasting, early in the morning. The person receiving the cure should not have eaten either: 'That's the way it used to be done years ago.' For health reasons, she no longer fasted and she would make the cure any time someone called by her home. She said, 'When I do it now, it seems to heal it as well.'

Her cure was popular; babies and adults regularly came for it. She recommended plenty of fresh air to ease the thrush and by the second visit she thought an improvement should be noticed. Occasionally she cured women of vaginal thrush using the same method as for oral thrush, breathing three times into their mouth for three days. Other people with this cure told me that they had acquired it because their father was dead when they were born. This woman, now almost eighty, said that her father was alive at the time of her birth, but that she had never met him. Another woman in north Roscommon told me likewise, and she added that if the person was ever to meet their father the cure would be lost.

I had conversations as well with two middle-aged men who had this cure and lived in the same town. One was a painter and decorator by trade. He also breathed three times into the baby's mouth, blessing himself before and after. When the people had left, he said a few prayers, 'just everyday prayers, but I've never told anyone what they were'. His mother had instructed him to keep this part of the cure secret. Parents generally brought their child to his home the first time; he then found out where they lived and called to their house the following two days to make the cure: 'I get their address and I go to them ... especially if it is a baby.' He would not take money for his cure but he said, 'we do take a gift'. The 'gift' he explained was part of the cure tradition. The person receiving the cure (or the parent) must give something in return; it could be a little, inexpensive present.

The other man managed a corner grocery shop. He mostly helped babies, sometimes an adult. It just took a few minutes to make the cure; 'it's short and sweet ... If it is thrush, it won't fail ... the first night I do it, it should start clearing.' Many people called into his shop with the sick child and he said, 'If I get a quiet minute, I'd have it done.'

Patrick Logan recorded a cure for warts in *Ulster Folklife* (1965), which was 'to touch the coat of a man who has never seen his father, but great care must be taken to ensure that the owner of the coat is unaware of the contact'. An elderly man from a Limerick village told me that a child who was born after their father died had the cure for whooping cough. To make the cure they had to breathe on the ill person, before eating any food (known as the 'fasting breath'), seven mornings in a row. Jan De Vries wrote of an old Scottish whooping cough cure, which was to 'Cut three small bunches of hair from the crown of the head of the child that has never seen its father.' The hair was then sewn into an unbleached rag and hung around the neck of the sick child.

Zora Neale Hurston, novelist, anthropologist and folklorist, is one of the most famous African-American women writers of the 1920–50 period. Against all the odds she produced a great quantity of work, including folklore collected from poor black communities in the south-east of the USA (particularly Florida). I was intrigued to see that for external ailments she had documented that, 'Persons of posthumous birth may cure any of these by simply blowing three times upon the affected area, saying after the first breath "In the name of the Father", after the second "And in the name of the Son", and after the third "And the Holy Ghost, A-men".'

# Breech Birth

A belief exists in the healing tradition of Ireland that those who are born breech (bottom or feet first) will have a back cure. Dr Blake called a child born in this way a 'footling'; he said they were bound to be a wanderer, and that they 'can cure lumbago by trampling on the patient's back, a rough and ready form of massage'. There was a healer (already discussed) in Roscommon who was known for her cure of back pain. To help the problem she would put her foot on the person's back and bless their spine. She had this cure because she was born breech; 'I have special healing for the back ... anyone that's a breech birth has the cure of the pain in the back.' Ted Kaptchuk and Michael Croucher investigated the healing arts' tradition worldwide, and they have written that, 'The most common folk technique, practised from Spain to Russia, was back-walking; fraught with ritual, this simple method of massaging the spine with the feet was usually conducted by a woman.'

In rural south Sligo I interviewed an eighteen-year-old with a cure for a bad back, 'bad backs ... pulled or strained ... I can't cure discs.' She was a breech birth and therefore has this cure. Her grandmother had told her mother that the child would be 'a blessing from God ... her feet are blessed, she'll have the cure of the bad back'. This young woman felt her cure was 'unusual but good'; she saw it as 'a gift ... it was meant to be ... I love doing it.'

To make the cure she explained, 'I'd get you to lie down on the ground and I'd stand up on your back ... say a prayer, and then get off, and that happens three days in a row.' The cure was made in the living room of her family home and she asked people to lie face down on the carpet. She would be alone with the person and she said, 'you can't be distracted by anything', you have to be 'focused on it [the cure], thinking about it and about the person as well ... You really want them to be better.' She would wear socks or go barefoot, and 'I tend to use my right [foot].' 'Before I step up, I make the shape of a cross [with] my foot over their back.' She would then say a silent prayer as she was standing on the person's back. 'I just say, Dear God please make [their name] better.' This procedure was repeated the following two days to complete the cure.

Even though she was small and slight she did not put all of her weight on the person; instead she leant on the adjacent couch. As a child she used to walk up and down the injured back three times; as an adult she would stand on the part of the back where they said the problem was. 'Everyone says you seem awful light, but I don't think that I'm actually light, I think they feel me light.' The old belief was that as the cure is made, 'they get light as they stand on the person's back,' her mother added.

I also spoke to a man in his sixties with this cure; he too lived in south Sligo, in a small market town. He was born breech and said that the nurse present at his birth had told his parents about the cure of back pain; she had made the sign of the cross on his feet and thereby started his cure. He blessed himself to commence the cure, then 'I will walk on the patient's back in the sign of the cross ... three times.' Each time he walked he said a blessing. Afterwards he silently said some prayers which took about five minutes. 'I'll not talk to the person until I've said the prayers.' 'I do say the Our Father, the Hail Mary, and the Glory ... and I always say, "If it's God's Will", I'll be the channel of curing this person's pain.'

He would only partially put his weight on the individual while leaning on two chairs either side of them. Those receiving the cure did not have to pray and they remained fully clothed. The cure was repeated on two other days, and so the ritual of walking on the back and saying the blessing took place a total of nine times. He did not accept money for the cure, but he believed that 'something has to pass [be given]'. 'In the old days it was tea or sugar, if they want to buy me a packet of biscuits.' This man had a lot of faith in his cure. 'I've seen people ... years in severe pain, I've seen them come and them bent, and I've seen them cycling home.' He was a gentle person, who said that often when he was making his cure, 'I get very calm ... for about five or ten minutes ... I do have a feeling of peace.'

## Same Surname Marriage

When a woman and man who have the same surname marry in Ireland, it was traditionally believed that they acquired a cure for whooping cough. This belief varies from place to place. A number of people told me that it is the children of these unions that have the cure of whooping cough, or shingles or mumps; one person felt that only the eldest son of the couple would have a cure. A full-time healer said that her parents had had the same surname and that some people thought this was why she was able to heal. Variations among my interviewees relating to this category of cure acquisition are discussed below.

## Whooping Cough

In a seaside town in County Sligo there was a woman who was an artist and she had a cure for whooping cough. This is a disease that is highly infectious and potentially life-threatening. Her cure came into existence forty-four years previously when she married a man with the same surname as her own, 'and they were waiting to queue up for the cure' when she arrived home from her honeymoon. Local people showed her how to make the cure. Initially she did not believe in it, 'but it worked always ... then I had to believe it'. Her husband was also eligible to make this cure, 'but he's never tried it out'.

She primarily helped young children, 'two-, three-, four-year-olds'. To make her cure she had to share food and drink with the child. 'I give them biscuits and a drink of orange ... I take some of it [the biscuit] and

I drink the orange ... from the same cup.' It could be any type of food or drink. 'I ask them what they like ... it might be an apple ... I've often given them chocolate.' It was crucial to the success of the cure that they ate and drank the same items, 'and I finish it if they don't finish it ... that is part of the cure'. She had learnt from experience how to make her cure most effectively. 'Some of them won't touch it after me having it and I've learned ... to drink it in the kitchen [privately] before giving it to them.' If the cure was for an infant, 'I just give the baby [a little] milk in a bottle ... I have to partake also; I take a sip of it ... He or she has got to drink that in my presence.' She said, 'I pray for them ... my own prayers ... I usually say it every day ... before sundown.'

The toddler had to be brought to her three times, only on Mondays and Thursdays, consecutively, and between sunrise and sunset. Following the first visit the child could be quite sick, but by the second one 'they are getting better' and she stressed that they must come the third time to finish off the cure and the whooping cough. She felt that people needed to have faith in the cure for it to be successful, and that in the past those cures that did not work, 'I knew it was because the parents didn't believe it.'

This cure was popular, but less so in recent years; she thought that most babies are now vaccinated against it. In 2015 there were 117 cases of whooping cough in Ireland; however, in 1953 when the vaccine was first introduced that figure was almost 5,000. She accepted no money but was sometimes given gifts, 'a box of chocolates ... most of them give nothing ... A thank you, that's all I wanted.' The cure was a positive part of this woman's life: 'You get such satisfaction and gratitude ... that you are able to do something like that, it's wonderful.'

I talked to a married couple who lived in the Ox Mountains of west Sligo; they too had a whooping cough cure because their surnames were the same. These people rarely made their cure, but were willing to do so if asked. The sick child had to visit them three times and bring a soft drink each time. They both drank a small amount of the liquid and the child drank the remainder; all three of them drank from the same container.

Logan documented a similar cure for whooping cough in 1963: 'collect the first and last piece of the breakfast food of a wife whose maiden name was the same as her married name. To this must be added the first and last piece of the husband's breakfast, and these are given to the child.' He has also written that in the past whooping cough claimed the lives of babies and young children in Ireland and that it caused deep distress to parents, which 'would account for the large number of cures which are still used' for this disease.

## Mumps

I interviewed a woman in her late forties living in a wild, majestic glen in north Leitrim. She had a mumps cure due to the fact that her parents had the same surname. Those who wanted the cure generally came to her home; it could be made any time and only one visit was necessary. She took the person a short distance from her house to a stream. 'I bring them down to the running stream ... the stream has to come from the mountain ... I put a rope in the shape of a halter around their neck and lead them to the water.' While they were wearing the halter she gave them three teaspoons of water from the stream to drink and they blessed themselves. She then said a prayer silently and asked the person to do likewise, 'any prayer they want to'. This ritual was performed twice more, and each time she walked the person away from the stream, then back to it to repeat the procedure: 'You lead them in and out [three times].'

She said that those who got the cure believed in it, even young people; 'nobody laughs', they all took it seriously. This woman had the cure from birth; however, she had just begun to use it two years prior to our meeting. She had relied on her brother to make it when required. A work colleague's daughter had mumps and she was asked to help. She raised the matter with her brother and he said to her, 'it's time you started', so she did. She wanted and accepted nothing for her cure. 'There's not many things in this world today that's for nothing … it didn't cost me anything to get the cure, so I'm not going to charge for it … just say a prayer for me.'

Also in County Leitrim, I spoke to a retired man who had a small farm and a comparable cure. He too had this cure because his mother had the same surname as his father, but in his area, it was the eldest son of the marriage that had a cure, 'that's the tradition around here'. 'It was an old man that told me I had it and showed me how to do it; he done it with me as a child … he had it and he done it … When he died then people started coming to me.'

He brought the individual with the mumps to a place close to his home where there was 'three mairn [mearing] water'. This was where three people's lands met, in this case where 'three drains go into one'. There was a little, shallow stream that could be stepped across. He also put a (donkey's) halter on the person, and 'I bring them across it [the stream] … over and back three times.' Then he lifted water from the stream onto a spoon, he dipped his hand in this water and made the sign of the cross on the person's neck with his wet hand, and he said a blessing. He had to repeat the blessing three times, making the sign of the cross on a different part of the neck each time, at either side and in the centre (front) of the neck. To end the cure, he prayed silently by the stream, 'an Our Father and three Hail Marys'.

This man had been assisting people for more than fifty years. It had been a well-utilised cure, but gradually the demand had decreased with the rise in childhood vaccination. An immunisation programme for mumps commenced in 1988. When I spoke to him he was making his cure mostly for older people; they were not vaccinated against it. Many of those who came for his cure had already been with a doctor and he said, 'I advise them to stay on their medication.'

He felt it was important to continue all aspects of the cure as it was taught to him; 'it's what you were learnt to believe in ... and when you believe in something you stick to it'. He thought that the traditional cures were very old, that they had been 'handed down from generation to generation ... [and] a lot of them came from pagan times'. His own cure could be traced back 'over a hundred years'. He was a caring man, and he told me that to 'do good for somebody, it gives you satisfaction ... while you carry on the tradition'.

O'Farrell recorded a mumps cure which was to, 'Bring the patient to a mearing where three townlands meet.' Alternatively, the sick person could wear a donkey halter and be led to a south flowing river, where they must drink the water 'without using any utensils'. Mac Coitir referred to an eighteenth-century Irish herbal book which 'recommended "foxglove and figwort gathered between the two feasts of St John (29 June or 4 July), boiled in the water of three boundaries" as a cure for a child who got fits or spasms while asleep'.

Lady Gregory retold the story of a young man who had become suddenly unwell and Biddy Early was consulted: 'And she gave him two bottles, the one he was to bring to a boundary water and to fill it up, and that was to be rubbed to the back, and the other was to drink ... She bid the boy to bring whatever was left of it to a river, and to pour it away with the running water.' Dr Logan speculated that by leading the sick person to flowing water and getting them to drink it 'may be an effort to transfer the disease to the water'. He wrote too that, 'The use of running water to carry away evil is very old and is found in the Saxon leechbooks.'

## Shingles

There was a woman (in her early fifties) with a cure for shingles in the south Donegal countryside. She was reluctant to tell me too much about how she made her cure, but she did say that she had to touch the person, that both parties had to pray, and that this healing ritual was repeated for three consecutive days. The person was asked to avoid wetting the shingles over the three days and for a few days afterwards. This woman acquired the cure as a consequence of her parents having the same surname. Her mother, from County Offaly, had this cure as well because her parents had had the same surname. Every time she made the cure she thought of her late mother. 'I always say, "Look Mam ... will you help me cure these people".' She believed that she was able to pass on her cure to all of her children.

I met a man in the north-west who also had a shingles cure; he was a builder and part-time farmer. He gave people a little jar of cream to rub on the affected area, 'once or twice a day ... there's enough in that for a week to ten days ... the pain goes straight away'. There were prayers associated with this cure. The cream was mainly a spreadable vegetable 'butter' to which he had done something; this was a secret. The man who gave him the cure had used a block of vegetable fat, but it was slow to soften on the skin.

He said that the cream was 'just a carrier for me ... you could use anything'. This man believed that others could prepare the cure as he did and it would not be effective; 'it won't cure unless you've been given the cure'. He received the cure from an elderly neighbour, a man he had worked with. The man was in poor health and one day he said to him, 'I'm giving you the cure ... that's it ... you have it now ... he showed me how to make it up.' This old man was well-known for the shingles cure and was entitled to make it as his parents had the same surname. He did not have children so he passed it to his young friend, and even though they were not related the cure had survived.

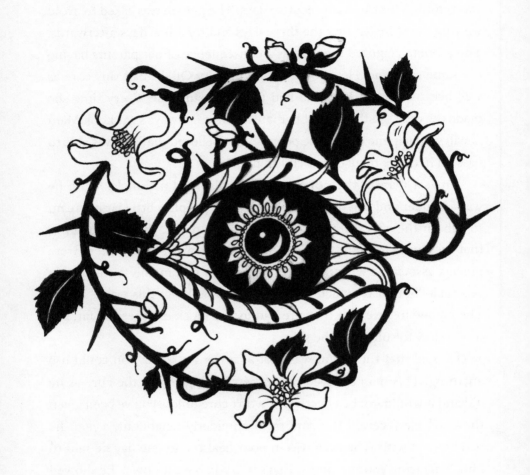

*Lady Wilde recorded, in 1888, a cure for a stye on the eyelid, which was to point a gooseberry thorn at it nine times and say, 'Away, away, away!'*

CHAPTER 11

# RITUAL

# Secrecy, Healing Days, Transference and Number

ITUAL IS AN IMPORTANT PART of most traditional Irish cures. It reinforces the unique identity of each cure. It also enhances the experience of those both giving and receiving cures, and can contribute towards the success of a cure. My research found that the ritual associated with cures incorporates a number of components, including secrecy, special healing days, the concept of transference and powerful numbers.

## Secrecy

Lots of cures contain an element of secrecy, about how the cure is made, the prayers that are said, the herbs that are used. When I asked people why their cure involved a secret, they usually replied that they did not know why, but that this was the tradition and it was important to adhere to it. Many believed that it would be detrimental to the cure to reveal the secret. For some the secrecy surrounding their cure is seen as a way of ensuring its protection and survival; they will not tell anyone how they make their cure until they are ready to pass it on.

From his research in Northern Ireland Anthony Buckley became aware that, 'Most people who have a cure will not tell its secret even to their spouse or closest relatives except in order to pass it on ... it is a common complaint that cures are disappearing because a man who dies suddenly may carry his secret to the grave.' Patrick Logan wrote that the 'fairy doctors' of previous centuries 'were careful to keep secret their knowledge of herbs, because knowledge which is secret is more effective' and he believed that, 'Any form of medicine is the better for its air of mystery and its ritual.' The secrecy aspect of the cure tradition may have links as well to the hereditary physicians of the Gaelic chieftains (pre-1600s), who closely guarded medical knowledge within their families.

Among the cures I investigated there are numerous examples of secrets, such as in this elderly man's cure for jaundice. He had made the cure for decades and it was in his family for generations. As a child his mother taught him how to make it and she told him to keep the essential ingredient secret. All he could say was that he had to go into the garden and dig up ninety herbs, counting them in bundles of thirty, and every thirtieth herb he threw away while saying a blessing. The herbs were then boiled in milk for a while, strained, bottled and stored in a fridge. He felt that if his cure was not kept secret, 'everyone could help themselves [to it] ... and if all knew, it would disintegrate'.

## Healing Days

Many traditional cures are made over three days, which are most commonly Mondays and Thursdays, and between sunrise and sunset.

It is generally believed that if these conditions are not met the cure will fail. Why can some Irish cures only be made after sunrise and before sunset? I have not come across an answer to this question from either those I interviewed or in the literature relating to cures. I suggest that it is because day is the time of light (culturally and spiritually associated with good, positivity and clarity of vision), whereas night is the time of dark (associated with evil, negativity and fear of the unseen); daylight would therefore have been perceived as more conducive to healing.

On a practical level, electricity did not come to many of the homes of rural Ireland until the 1950s, so in the past people's lives were dictated by the seasons. They rose with the dawn, worked with the light, and retired indoors or to bed with the dusk. It would have made sense for a person to visit a house and receive a cure during daylight hours. In addition, transport was limited, with most people primarily walking or cycling up to the 1960s, activities hindered by darkness.

Why are Monday and Thursday linked to lots of cures? Again, I have not found an obvious answer, but as a result of my research, I have drawn the following conclusion. From the mid-1800s (post Famine) to the close of the twentieth century Ireland has been a deeply religious, predominantly Roman Catholic, society. Sunday was a day of rest, a day to go to Mass and to spend with family. All unnecessary work was to be avoided and that probably included making a cure. Cures could be started on Monday and three days later, Thursday, made again, and concluded after three more days (excluding Sunday) on Monday. Most cures can also be commenced on Thursday, and repeated the following Monday and Thursday.

A woman who had a toothache cure told me that in the late 1960s she brought her young daughter, with severe eczema, for a cure in rural north Leitrim. She had to bring butter to the woman who made the cure and this was mixed with herbs. The cure consisted of three little balls of herbal butter and she was instructed to rub one butter ball each day on the child's eczema. It was important to do this over newspaper and any bits of butter or skin which fell onto the paper were to be burned. She had to make three consecutive visits, Monday, Thursday and Monday, to collect the herbal butter and was given three balls each time, nine butter balls altogether, to be applied over a nine-day period. This cure could not be made on Sunday and no herbal butter was to be rubbed on the child's eczema that day. 'It worked, it got completely cured,' she remembered.

## Transference

In Irish folk medicine the concept of transference is based on the belief that ill health can be passed from the affected person or animal to something or somebody else. Meda Ryan, in her book on Biddy Early, alludes to the notion of transference. She wrote that 'very often ... her power in curing meant the transference of the sickness to some other living creature ... She took the evil off the servant boy and put it on the horse once more. When the man went home the horse was dead.' Lady Wilde documented a cure for mumps in the late nineteenth century which was to, 'Wrap the child in a blanket, take it to the pigsty, rub the child's head to the back of a pig, and the mumps will leave it and pass from the child to the animal.' Logan recorded an old ulcer cure from Connemara (Galway) in which the patient had to be completely buried in earth; this was he said 'an example of pagan magic in which the disease is transferred to the earth, which is the great healer and purifier. Such transference cures are found in folk medicine everywhere.'

There are many cures for warts in the Irish healing tradition and they often employ the concept of transference. Nora Smyth was told of a wart cure by a teenage girl in Armagh, 'I had a really ugly wart on my eyelid and my mum cut the potato in half, rubbed it on my eyelid and buried it. When the potato had rotted my wart had gone.' Another cure for warts was to leave a stone or a small potato at a crossroads, and it was believed that whoever picked it up would pick up the warts too. I met a man in north Clare who recalled that when he was a boy in the 1970s, he had developed three big warts on his hand. During a visit to his grandmother, she asked him had he found any coins along the road. He replied that there were three coins lying together on the road and that he had happily put them in his pocket. The wise old woman laughed and explained to her grandson that he had picked up more than money. To rid the lad of the warts, she rubbed each with a coin and directed him to lay the three coins on a road, touching each other. The next unfortunate person to pick up this money would also acquire the warts, and so it came to pass; within a short time his warts had disappeared.

A man with a cure for gallstones told me that in the 1980s the warts on his hand had been cured by an elderly local man. The man touched the warts with two rushes and said some prayers. He then crumpled up one rush and on the second rush he tied a knot for each wart. This rush had to be buried in soft earth, and he explained that as the rush rotted and vanished so too would the warts; they did. Dr Logan thought that, 'These methods of transferring, washing and wasting warts are probably thousands of years old.'

In south Cavan, a cure for epilepsy was described to me. A hole must be drilled in the wall or ground wherever the first epileptic attack took place. A piece of fingernail or hair should be taken from the sick person, wrapped in paper, put in the hole and sealed. This must be done in secret by someone who witnessed the seizure. Every day they must pray for the person to remain free of epilepsy, one Hail Mary, Our Father and Glory Be. However, if they forgot to say these prayers for more than three days, the condition would return. O'Farrell documented an epilepsy cure which was to bury 'a tress of the patient's hair and his nail clippings while saying a prayer: By the power of Mary and the soul of Paul, let the great illness lie in the clay forever'.

I talked to a woman who had cures for shingles and piles; the latter one was looked for infrequently. She used a branch from the 'boot' tree (elder) to make it. Taking part of the branch, she cut it into several cross sections; the elder is easy to cut as it is soft and pithy inside. She sewed the pieces of wood into a small cloth pouch and instructed people to 'wear it or carry it in their wallet ... their pocket'. This woman said that as the tree sections broke down and disappeared, the piles went also; 'as it goes into powder ... the piles then gradually go'.

In Irish folklore the elder was associated with witchcraft, and Mac Coitir has written that, 'The elder is a dark, feminine, witch's tree possessing great healing powers.' He referred to an old English (Suffolk) cure; the belief was 'that elder sticks kept in the pocket would prevent saddle sores when riding'. Allen and Hatfield found that the elder was 'one of the most widely used of all British and Irish folk herbs ... this tree's employment in a salve for burns and scalds has been recorded very widely in Ireland'. Logan recalled that garlands woven from sprigs of elder or rowan trees were placed on the lid of the churn, to protect the butter from the fairies or bad neighbours.

I had an interesting conversation with a man in north Cavan who made a cure for hernia, 'hiatus hernia or the ordinary hernia'. He was in his early forties, a farmer, mechanic and father. He understood that most of the people (adults and children) who looked for the cure had already been diagnosed and were hoping to avoid surgery. His cure entailed an unusual and secret ritual, and could only be made in summertime during the growing season. Those that came for this cure brought a handmade hay rope with them. In the past ropes like this were common in rural Ireland being used to tie down cocks of hay in the fields. These days he said, 'a lot of people don't understand what it is' and it could be challenging for them to get one. His wife normally took phone enquiries and she explained about the rope.

'[The] person has to bring a rope of about twenty foot, a hay rope, and I bring them to a place where there's ash trees, and I do it [the cure] on the ash tree.' He made the cure on Mondays and Thursdays, and arranged for people to arrive in the evening when he was home from work. 'I try to have everyone at the house at the one time.' Then he took them to an area nearby where there were many ash trees. They had to wait at a distance as he brought each person individually to a tree. This man would not reveal exactly how he made the cure, but he did say that he used a different tree for each person, that the cure took twenty minutes to make and the hay rope 'stays at the tree'. To complete the cure, he had to say some prayers whenever it suited him, 'that evening … a week later … maybe driving along in the van'.

He believed that the person would be cured 'when the tree knits back together … and the rope rots away … the end of the summer you'd find a [positive] change'. It was as if the ailment had been transferred to the hay rope and the tree, and that as the person's handmade rope decayed and the tree healed, so did their hernia. This cure was part of his family's life; 'people calling to the door for the cure … it was just part of what happened here every summer'. He was a generous man, and even though he was very busy with the cure during the summer months, he said, 'it's nice to do something … to help somebody out … it didn't do me any bad … I was lucky since I took it on.'

In 1931 Harriet Hunt, from the Isle of Man, recounted a story about a cure for a 'protrusion' performed on a baby boy in her care in the early 1890s in Donegal. On May morning before sunrise 'wee Harry' was taken to the top of a hill, and there 'the old woman split a willow-wand sufficiently to allow the child to be passed through the hoop'. As the sun rose, they passed the infant through the opening three times, saying a blessing each time 'then carefully bound together [the tree] with scarlet wool. As the young wood knit together the child's wound would heal.'

Niall Mac Coitir describes the ash as a 'sacred Guardian Tree', as being connected with healing and fertility, and 'a symbol of the well-being of the land itself'. He recalled that, 'In England children with ruptures were passed through an ash split held open by wedges of oak. The ash was then bandaged up and as the split healed so the child was cured.' Patrick Logan noted that some English folk cures for whooping cough involved 'passing the child through a hole in a stone or through a split tree ... All these are examples of an effort to pass the disease on to something else.'

## Number

Three, nine, seven and five are the numbers closely associated with Irish cures. Why are these numbers so important? The answer is elusive and multi-layered. Their use is deliberate and very old, possibly thousands of years. It has been affected by religious belief, political power and societal values. These three ever-present influences have responded to events (dramatic and subtle) which have taken place over millennia. This is an area worthy of greater study from a variety of perspectives, particularly with regard to the significance of these numbers in other countries. My analysis has focused on the way in which they are utilised in cures and healing ritual in Ireland today, and on references I found to them in related literature.

## Three

Three is the most powerful and prevalent number in traditional Irish cures. I consulted Sligo wood carver Michael Quirke, who told me that in many cultures odd numbers are viewed as female; three, five, seven and nine are all odd numbers. His carvings are rooted in mythology, and he explained that in ancient Irish belief there were three aspects to the Goddess, Virgin, Mother and Old Woman (the life cycle). He viewed the triple spiral symbol as representing woman, her breasts and womb, and each spiral is a serpent, the symbol of the goddess and the pre-Christian religion.

A beautiful triple spiral has been carved on the huge stone which guards the opening to Newgrange passage tomb in the Boyne Valley, County Meath. Now a World Heritage Site, Brú na Bóinne consists of three great burial mounds, Knowth, Dowth and Newgrange. At dawn of the winter solstice, 21 December, the shortest day of the year, light from the rising sun shines through a gap in the stones (the roof-box) at the entrance to Newgrange. As the sun strengthens a beam of light moves along the passageway to illuminate the womb-like burial chamber within. Professor John Waddell writes of this solar phenomenon 'it has been calculated that at the time the tomb was built 5000 years ago, the beam of sunlight would have bisected the chamber and illuminated a triple spiral carved on ... the end recess'. This annual 'return of the sun' must have been momentous for our ancestors, bringing with it hope, and the promise of new growth and life.

The Tuatha Dé Danann had three goddesses who personified Ireland, Éiru, Banba and Fodla, and the first of these deities has given her name to our modern Republic, Éire. Proinsias Mac Cana has written that the 'concept of threeness' was highly significant for the Celts, and 'It has been observed that triplication may have an intensifying force and that it may also convey the concept of totality.' Poet, novelist and Irish mythology scholar Robert Graves, in his 1948 classic tome *The White Goddess*, spoke of the three members of her 'moon-trinity ... the New Moon is the white goddess of birth and growth; the Full Moon, the red goddess of love and battle; the Old Moon, the black goddess of death and divination'.

In Christianity the male God has three aspects, Father, Son and Holy Spirit, known collectively as the Trinity. The Trinity is an important feature of many contemporary Irish cures, as a blessing often accompanies a cure. A Tyrone man made a heart fever cure using three arm measurements, in conjunction with three blessings which included the individual's name: 'I'm doing the person's name in the Trinity ... the Trinity is a blessing on its own.' He repeated the cure three weeks later for those who had this problem. 'I have to check it in three weeks ... Jesus laid in a tomb for three days ... the whole thing comes through him.'

If you drive (especially in autumn and spring) through the spectacular mountain valley of Glencar on the Sligo/Leitrim border, you will see a gigantic, three-pointed symbol on the side of Tor Mór hill. It was cleverly and painstakingly constructed in the 1980s by planting contrasting trees of golden larch and evergreen spruce, and it is known as the Trinity Knot. Niamh Mac Cabe, whose father Jim created this impressive sight, describes the ancient symbol as representing 'the united elements of humanity: body, mind, and spirit. The continuous intertwining bands represent the impenetrable endlessness of eternity.'

Professor Emyr Estyn Evans of Queen's University, Belfast, recorded in 1957, that 'the Midsummer fires still burn strongly in some country districts ... To walk three times sunwise round the fire was to ensure a year without sickness' and that, 'A glowing turf from the fire was carried three times sunwise round the dwelling house.' From Scotland, Janet and Colin Bord highlighted the tradition of pregnant women going sunwise (clockwise) three times around a church to ensure an easy birth 'and boats would row around sunwise three times before starting their journey'. Padraic O'Farrell noted a traditional cure for seasickness which was to put three drops of sea water on the baby's tongue before it was baptised. This 'would give it lifelong immunity from seasickness'.

Tobar na mBan Naomh (Well of the Holy Women) is located on the rugged coastline of south-west Donegal. This little holy well overlooks the safe waters of Teileann Bay, close to the Slieve League cliffs. In the eighth century, or earlier, Christian monks reputedly sailed from here to Iceland. The well is dedicated to three holy women, known as Ciall, Tuigse, *agus* Náire (Sense, Understanding and Modesty), who lived and are buried locally. Tradition says that they were the sisters of St Colmcille; more likely they were three pre-Christian goddesses. In his writings on this well Joseph Szövérffy alluded to 'the Celtic cult of three Goddesses ... the Mothers' across many European countries (in particular Germany), who were 'often associated with water, springs, and wells'. There are three smooth, rounded 'curing stones' at a simple 'altar' nearby and those with ailments rub them on the parts of their body in need of healing. Pilgrimage to this holy well takes place on 23 June, Bonfire Night, the celebration of midsummer.

A short distance west of Teileann, in the heart of the Donegal Gaeltacht (Irish-speaking area), is the valley of Gleann Cholm Cille. On the slopes of the lush, green hill above the village, with panoramic views of the Atlantic Ocean beyond, a small holy well is perched. A high, long, L-shaped ridge of stones surrounds the well and a grassy path leads through this cairn to the water in a cool, dark alcove. The holy well and indeed the whole valley is named in honour of Colmcille. Professor Michael Herity documented the annual *turas* (journey) which circles this glen, visits the holy well, involves fifteen stations (prayer and movement ritual) and takes over three hours to complete. He wrote of 'the many pilgrims who have visited the well since antiquity, each carrying up three stones, which they place on the cairn, one for each of the three circuits, saying the prescribed prayers'. Also, 'The pilgrim drinks from the well here having first thrown out three drops of water in the name of the Trinity.'

## Cures Made in Threes

I was intrigued to be told by a number of my interviewees that they often make their cure in threes. A woman with a sprain cure, who had been helping people for fifty years, had noticed that three people usually come for the cure close to each other. 'The funny part about the cure of the sprain is when I make it for one, I make it for three, and I mightn't make it for a month ... then as sure as one comes, two more will come ... I've noticed that over the years ... and that's amazing!'

Likewise, the man who had a Bell's Palsy cure, for thirty-six years, had observed that if he made one cure, it would shortly be followed by two more requests for the cure. 'Once I start one, I'll get three ... It comes that way in threes ... very strange ... all the time. I could bet my house on it!'

## Nine

Nine is an important number in the healing tradition of Ireland. Logan has written that the 'use of the number nine is very primitive ... is part of the ancient leech lore of the Irish and is often found in modern folk medicine'. He recalled that it was laid down in an old law, that the patient's wounds 'must be examined by a doctor on the ninth day after an injury'. A man with a bleeding cure said that the traditional belief was that it took nine days to heal a wound or knit a bone, another nine days to get strong, and a further nine days to be fully healed.

Peter Kavanagh knew of an epilepsy cure which was, 'Nine one-inch pieces of elder twig, formed into a necklace with three strands of silk thread, and tied around the neck'. He referred to a cure for mumps: 'Put the winkers of an ass' on the sick person, and lead them in and out of a pigsty nine times, while saying, 'Let the pigs take the mumps away.' A blacksmith could lay a terrible curse by going naked to his forge before dawn for nine consecutive days, turning the anvil nine times, and hitting it three times after each turn. Kavanagh was convinced that 'no earthly power can neutralise any curse of his'.

Niall Mac Coitir noted a love charm: 'It was believed that if a girl placed nine leaves of yarrow under her pillow while saying a charm, she would dream of her future husband that night.' Lady Wilde wrote in 1888 that, 'If you walk nine times around a fairy rath at the full of the moon, you will find the entrance.' She recorded a cure for a stye on the eyelid which was to point a gooseberry thorn at it nine times and to say, 'Away, away, away!' Some children I was teaching in rural south Sligo in 2000 told me of an equivalent cure for a stye. This entailed picking ten gooseberry thorns, pointing nine of them at (but not touching) the infected eye, saying a blessing, and then tossing the tenth thorn over the left shoulder. Dr Heraughty believed this cure was possibly linked to the very old practice of lancing a stye with a gooseberry thorn.

In Irish legend the Salmon of Knowledge lived in a pool which was the source of the River Boyne, named in honour of goddess Bóinn, mother of Aengus (god of love). The pool was surrounded by nine sacred hazel trees; the salmon had eaten nuts from these trees and consequently acquired complete wisdom. Finnéigeas, the druid, spent seven years trying to catch this fish, but when he finally did his servant boy Fionn was first to taste it, and thereby became destined to be a great warrior, hero and seer. In Ireland the salmon is linked to good health and there is a saying, *Sláinte an Bhradáin Chugat*, which translates as, 'Health of the Salmon to You'.

The royal palace of pre-Christian Ulster was at Emain Macha, near Armagh. A story is told of Macha being forced to race the king's horses when heavily pregnant, because of a boast by her foolish husband. She won the race and as she finished gave birth to twins, then died. However, before she took her last breath, she placed a curse upon the men of Ulster for nine generations; that at times of greatest need, when they were under attack, they would be weak and defenceless, and suffer the pains of childbirth.

*Over Nine Waves* is the title of Marie Heaney's book of legends, and it refers to the arrival from northern Spain of the Milesians and the Gaels, who overthrew the Tuatha Dé Danann and took control of Ireland. 'We will go back to our boats and retreat from the shore over the distance of nine waves. Then we will come back over the nine waves, disembark and take this land by force if need be.' Professor Mac Cana wrote that the 'ninth wave' would have constituted 'a magic boundary' for the Celts.

Máire MacNeill, writing about Mount Brandon in west Kerry, noted that:

> There is a tradition that in the old days the turas (pilgrimage) was made at dawn ... The 'rounds' consisted of praying at the ruined oratory and then encircling it and the pillar-stone and the 'graves' nine times while saying the Rosary, and ended by taking a drink from the well ... those who hoped for a cure for backache stood with their backs against the pillar-stone.

The number nine played a key role in some of the cures I explored, such as in the one made by an elderly countrywoman for pain in the back and sprain. If the injured person or animal (cow, horse or dog) was not physically present she simply prayed for them, but if they came to her, she prayed and touched them. She made the sign of the cross using her right thumb over the damaged area while saying the secret cure prayer. She repeated this ritual nine times.

I interviewed a woman with a thrush cure. She had to breathe into the person's mouth three times and repeat this ritual for three days in a row. She explained that it took nine days to make a cure; 'every cure is nine days', that was the old belief. 'It's coming on the person three days before they come to me, and then it's three days for me to do it, and three days is the complete thing getting better, that's the ninth day.' A seventh son who cured ringworm made it over three days too. He said that if the problem was severe people might have to come back for another cure; he never made the cure twice, only once or three times;

'It's three or nine [days], I don't know why ... if it's very bad, then it is going to take nine times.'

## Seven

The number seven is and has been important to traditional cures, and religious belief and ritual in Ireland. It is most obviously associated with the tradition of the seventh daughter/son having special healing power. Dr Blake remarked that 'in all lands and ages three and seven and their multiples have been looked on as mystic numbers'. Bob Quinn understands that the number seven indicates 'perfection or holiness'. One seventh son faith healer told me that 'seven is a significant number in the Bible'. It is written in this holy book that God created the world in seven days and that on the seventh day he rested.

Archaeologist Marion Dowd refers to a cave on the pilgrimage island of Lough Derg, that may have provided inspiration for a fourteenth-century Italian fresco 'which depicts St Patrick overlooking the entrance to purgatory – represented as a cave with seven chambers each containing one of the seven deadly sins'. Environmentalist David Hickie tells us that under Brehon Law (before the mid-1600s), there were seven very important and protected trees in Ireland; known as the 'chieftains', they were oak, hazel, holly, yew, ash, pine and apple. Lady Wilde recalled that in the Irish healing tradition there existed 'seven herbs of great value and power; they are ground ivy, vervain, eyebright, groundsel, foxglove, the bark of the elder-tree, and the young shoots of the hawthorn'.

Seven smooth, round stones can be found at the Angel's Well (Tobar na nAingeal) in the Donegal hills. Those who are making the station of this holy well are directed to move each stone around their body three times. They must also walk around the altar and the two small wells seven times, saying a decade of the Rosary each time. When I visited the well in 2006, I got a leaflet there detailing the station. Five Our Fathers, five Hail Marys, one Creed and one Gloria were to be said on both sides of the two wells. But an account of this holy well recorded by Sarah Kelly nearly seventy years earlier (part of The Schools' Collection), stated that the station prayers were seven Our Fathers, seven Hail Marys and seven Glory Bes. She documented that the pilgrimage took place on May Eve, and that people hoped to be cured of their aches and pains (NFCS 1096: 175).

In 2017 I walked up to Mám Éan holy well on a lonely mountain pass near Recess in Connemara. Almost twenty years before me writer Elizabeth Healy had joined a local community pilgrimage to this well. She talked to those present, and observed their movements and prayers. To perform the station, people had to walk seven times around each of the three original features (the holy well and the two ruined, circular, stone 'beds') and say three prayers for every round, one Our Father, Hail Mary, and Glory Be.

As pilgrims climb the holy mountain of Croagh Patrick in west Mayo they come upon a small cairn of stones, Leacht Beanáin (Benin's Grave). They must walk clockwise around this station seven times, praying as they move, seven Our Fathers, seven Hail Marys, and one Creed. There are two other stations in this pilgrimage, Leaba Phádraig (Patrick's Bed) on the windswept summit, and Reilig Mhuire (Mary's Graveyard) which consists of three small cairns and is sited a short distance below on the western slope. The same ritual of prayer and movement is repeated at each of the three stations.

MacNeill recounted the story of St Patrick and how he was encircled by 'demon-birds' on this mountain, so he threw his bell at them, and:

> they disappeared and came no more to Ireland for seven years, seven months, seven days and nights … [and] Patrick left seven of his household … to guard Ireland. [She wrote too that]

Reilig Mhuire ... before Christianity ... must have had another dedication, probably to a goddess ... a clash of religions and a struggle between a patriarchal and a matriarchal culture ... the victory of Christianity over Paganism.

## Five

Five is primarily linked to the prayers that are used in cures. Fifteen (five times three) is part of the healing tradition of Ireland as well. The number five was essential to the ritual attached to one man's heart and head cures; for both he had to say fifteen prayers, five Our Fathers, five Hail Marys and five Glory Bes. For his heart cure, he pressed a glass full of oatmeal to five parts of the body as he said a blessing. For the headache, he made the sign of the cross on the person's head five times to start and finish the cure.

The number five is a significant part of the station associated with some holy wells. At St Patrick's Well in Dromard, west Sligo, I found a laminated, typed page informing pilgrims how to make the station. The initial part of the procedure involves removing one's shoes, standing at the well, and saying five Our Fathers, five Hail Marys and one Creed. The same prayers are then said outside the wall surrounding the well and this ritual is repeated three times. Logan took note of the prescribed prayers for those who visit St Brigid's holy well near Liscannor, west Clare:

> they kneel at the modern statue of St Brigid and say five Paters, five Aves and five Glorias ... The pilgrims then climb some steps to the higher level and repeat the five Paters, Aves and Glorias ... The third praying place is an old stone cross up a slight incline ... here the prayers are repeated and the cross circled.

I believe that five was also an important pre-Christian number. St Brigid's Well, near the M7 motorway and Kildare town, is popular with the public. This is a manicured holy well in a peaceful and pastoral location. It has had a number of modern additions to the area around it, including walls, railings, altars, arches and a life-size, bronze statue of the saint. A very interesting aspect of this well is the presence of five stones, known as the 'prayer stones' and probably of pagan origin. These roughly cut stones (40 cm tall by 25 cm wide) are embedded in the ground at 5 m intervals. The well is to the rear of the site and the stones are placed in a line approaching it; they appear to be over the underground stream which flows from it.

On the day I was documenting this holy well, a Traveller couple arrived with their eight children, including a baby. They stayed for thirty minutes, engaging with all parts of the well site and continuously praying. The young mother touched her infant to each of the five stones. They blessed themselves with well water and finally tied one of the baby's vests to the adjacent rag tree. I spoke to the parents who told me that they were originally from this area, but now live in England. They were here to bless the new baby and all the family. They said that for years numerous women and men have come to this well looking for cures and blessings. A lot of people have great belief in this holy well, and in the power of Brigid to help and to heal.

St Brigid's Shrine at Faughart (allegedly her birthplace) is close to the hearts of many in the north-east. It is deep in the countryside, on high ground overlooking Dundalk and the Irish Sea, and a short distance from south Armagh. The setting is quite lovely; a small stream rushes through a glade of magnificent beech trees. At the centre of the elaborate station is the simple, white-walled, glass-enclosed shrine, above which there is a statue of Brigid. The holy site extends to an open field downhill, where five pre-Christian healing stones are located adjacent to the stream; they are part of the station ritual.

The stones vary in shape and size, and their appearance is reflective of their name, the hoof stone, the knee stone, the waist stone, the eye stone and the head stone. I was told by a local woman that all of these stones are used for healing and that for some the name dictates their cure. Those suffering from headaches press their head into the head stone, a rock in the field wall with a curved indentation around which a white circle has been painted. The eye stone is a small, circular depression where water collects; it is part of a big boulder which people lie upon as this rock has a reputation for curing back pain. The knee stone is possibly a double *ballán* stone and pilgrims kneel in its two depressions as they pray. Some sit on top of the waist stone; my informant thought it may have been used to assist with childbirth. The hoof stone lies beside the little stream; it is quite big, roughly square, lichen covered and it has the imprint of a giant horseshoe. These five healing stones are a thought-provoking mixture of pagan and Christian belief and practice.

With regard to literary sources, Niall Mac Coitir has written that, 'In ancient Ireland there were five great trees considered by legend to be sacred above all others ... All five stood at or near important royal or sacred sites.' Three of the trees were ash, at Tara, County Meath, Farbill and Uisneach, County Westmeath, an oak at Moone, County Kildare, and a yew at Old Leighlin, County Carlow. He also referred to five streams which flowed from a well at Mannanán Mac Lir's (the sea god's) royal fortress, and that this was 'the well of knowledge, and that the five streams represent the five streams through which knowledge go, i.e. the five senses'.

Ireland is divided into four provinces; Connacht to the west, Ulster to the north, Leinster to the east; and Munster to the south. However, in pre-Christian times there was a fifth territory incorporating fertile County Meath, with royal Tara at its centre. The word for province in Irish is *cúige*, meaning fifth. Mac Cana believed that it was the Fir Bholg tribe who divided the country into five, and that 'a fivefold conception of the world ... is more or less universal and is particularly well attested in India and China'.

Robert Graves was fascinated by the ancient Irish alphabet (ogham) in which each letter was named after the tree starting with that letter, for example, I, Idho, was yew. In this alphabet there were five vowels and he wrote, 'I take them to be the trees particularly sacred to the White Goddess, who presided over the year and to whom the number five was sacred.'

# CHAPTER 12

# The Process and Atmosphere

## The Process

WHEN SOMEONE NEEDS A CURE, a process must be gone through to get it; this process can be easy or difficult, depending on a number of factors. These include finding someone with the required cure, making contact and possibly meeting them, and the ritual attached to the cure. The ritual can be simple and quick, or complicated and time-consuming, with many variations in between. I believe that the process involved in getting a cure can contribute to a positive outcome; making a conscious decision to try a cure, locating, pursuing and committing to it, is proactive and empowering, and could help stimulate the person's innate healing ability.

Based on the replies I got from my interviewees, I have taken a closer look at the following elements of the process: the passing of information by word of mouth, the necessity of asking for a cure, and if the person seeking the cure has to be physically present or not. I have

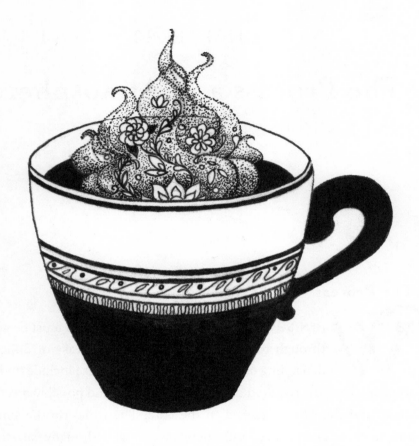

*Those with cures often make them in their homes. They welcome the people who come looking for their help; they listen to their problems and sometimes a cup of tea is shared.*

also examined the popularity of cures, where people come from (locals or strangers), and what type of people get cures.

## Word of Mouth

The majority of cures are located through word of mouth; this is an important aspect of the cure tradition in Ireland. If you need a particular cure, you let it be known, and between your friends, family, work colleagues and neighbours, a name or some helpful information will usually be found. Those with cures are generally very private about their cure. They will not publicise or advertise it; they need to be sought out, like the woman with a cure for mumps who told me that people hear of it by 'word of mouth, same way as you'. I had actually spent an afternoon trying to find her, as she lived well off the beaten track in the mountains of north Leitrim. She felt that people who want a cure should have to look for it and that this search is part of the cure; 'if they want me, they'll find me ... If you have belief, you'll travel any journey.'

I spoke to a man who made a cure for a foreign body in the eye and he thought that the details regarding his cure spread quickly in workplaces, like factories and building sites, where eye injuries occurred. 'If someone phones up and is cured, they'll mention it on' to the next person who needs it.

And there was a woman in east Leitrim who had a cure for orf in sheep which she made for hundreds of farmers every year. The farmers told each other of her cure, particularly when they met to sell their livestock. Her phone number was on public display in the agricultural supplies store in Sligo town, and one of her neighbours who worked there regularly recommended the cure. Also, I visited a busy mart in south Sligo to see a phone number for the orf cure painted on the wall there.

## Ask for a Cure

Some of the people I interviewed told me that if you want a cure, you must ask the person that has it to make it for you, ask for their help. They saw this belief as part of the cure tradition that has been handed down from previous generations. A man with a sprain cure recalled, 'I often heard ... older people saying ... people should hear about you from word of mouth.' He did not like to tell anyone that he had the cure or to offer to help them; 'I'd sooner you heard it off somebody, and came back and asked me.' Lady Wilde, writing in the 1880s about the cure for a 'fairy dart' (joint pain), said that a well-known fairy-woman was often called upon to help, but that 'she had no power unless asked to make the cure, and she took no reward at the time; not till the patient was cured'.

A few of those with cures felt that they could not tell people directly that they had the required cure, but they could tell someone connected to the person. The man with a Bell's palsy cure clarified, 'if I meet someone and they have Bell's palsy, I can't say to them, come to me and I'll do the charm'. However, he could tell the person they were with that he had this cure; 'there's my number, [you] tell them to ring me'. Many believed that they should not discuss their cure casually or carelessly, such as the man who had a cure for mumps; he understood that the old belief was that you must not talk about a cure unless you were going to get it, and to do so would be 'bad luck'.

## Physically Present or Not

Of my ninety-three interviewees the divide was more or less equal between those who said that the person wanting their cure had to be physically present to receive it, and those who could make their cure solo, entrust it to a third party to deliver, or post it. Having said this, some of the people in the former category made their cure without seeing the person, if that was the only option.

One healer told me that she sometimes tried to cure an individual who was not physically present, usually because they were in hospital. 'I bless something belonging to them ... and I get them to say the prayer.' For three days she repeated this ritual, as she would for those who came to her home. A seventh son faith healer said that he preferred to see people in person, but a few times he had posted a cure. 'An article would be sent to me by someone, and I would have treated it with holy water and sent it back to them.' He was reluctant to heal in this way though, as he felt the success rate could be diminished.

## Numbers and Where From

All of the people I interviewed had cures that were alive and well, and being utilised. However, their popularity varied; some cures were in demand several times a week, while others were made only a few times each year. Cures were generally known to those who lived locally to them and often within the broader, surrounding area (a particular part of a county). We live on an island and with regard to the traditional cures this means that a natural containment exists. Some people travel long distances (hundreds of kilometres) from their homes to other parts of Ireland and Northern Ireland in search of a cure. A number of my interviewees said that residents of other countries also avail of their cures, most notably from the UK and the USA, places with many people of Irish descent.

I spoke to a woman who made a well-known herbal cure for shingles. It had remained in the same Leitrim village for decades and people travelled from all over Ireland to get it. 'We make hundreds [of cures] ... and so many young people coming for it.' She had an arrangement with the local butcher whereby he kept her cures in his shop fridge (there was a small charge attached) and people could collect it there during business hours, 'just in case I wouldn't be here and someone is after travelling'. And a man with a herbal cure for gallstones told me that it had been in his family for more than forty years and that many, many people had taken it. It had gone south to Tipperary, north to Donegal, and east to England.

## Types of People

What type of people get cures? This was one of the questions I asked my interviewees and the reply was, invariably, all types. Women and men, old and young, rural and urban, working and middle class, Catholic and Protestant, and those without religion; there is no typical person who gets a traditional cure. A farmer in Kildare, who had a very popular cure which was used to help strokes, recalled that if he went away for a few days, 'the answer machine ... could have one hundred messages when you come back'. Every type of person got his cure; they were mostly strangers, of all ages, different religions, now and then nurses and lots of Travellers.

An elderly Leitrim woman had cures for foot rot, sprain and pain in the back. The latter two were better known and she made about one hundred cures per year. She helped animals and humans: children, teenagers, workmen, footballers and tug-of-war participants. Some people were local, many were strangers from the surrounding counties and Northern Ireland. She had phone requests for her cures from the USA too; 'it's amazing the way they know'.

## Travellers

The Traveller community is a small (about 33,000) but important part of Irish society. They are a traditional, nomadic people with a unique identity, and a rich culture and heritage. In 2017 Travellers were formally recognised by the state as a distinct ethnic group.

Many Travellers have a strong belief in cures and avail of them frequently. They also like to visit holy wells and to pray at them for blessings, good health and cures. At Killargue holy well in County Leitrim I found photographs of Traveller children at their Christening and Holy Communion ceremonies; their names were attached and the wish, 'Pray for us.' When I was documenting Tobernalt holy well, near Sligo town, two Traveller women arrived with children. They began to walk around this wooded area and to recite their prayers. I witnessed the older woman push her back into a curve in the Mass rock, which is known as a cure for back pain.

In *Pavee Pictures*, midst Derek Speirs' striking black and white photographs of the Traveller community, their experiences, beliefs and hopes are expressed. Kathleen from Dublin explained that, 'Travellers are very religious. I love a lot of blessed pictures and statues and plenty of holy water in the place. If I miss Mass it takes a lot out of me. Travellers believe a lot in priests and cures. We are very superstitious.'

## The Atmosphere

When someone gets a cure, the atmosphere is usually relaxed, friendly and positive. Those with cures often make them in their homes and they are welcoming to the people who come looking for their help. A significant human interaction occurs; an individual (non-professional) gives their personal cure to another individual. In many instances the sick person is made the centre of attention, their concerns are listened to and compassion is shown for their plight. As with most things Irish, there is generally a lengthy conversation attached to the procedure and sometimes a cup of tea. I believe that the atmosphere which surrounds the receiving of a cure can positively influence the outcome, that it can kick-start and strengthen the healing process.

I found the woman who made a whooping cough cure to be kind and generous. She recalled that occasionally after the cure was made the child's parents 'want to stay and talk, and they get comfort I think from being with me, knowing that it's good for their child'. Another person recounted a story of a neighbour who had called to see her late one night. This woman had a bad toothache and a lot of pain, 'So I sat her down and made a cup of tea, and I said the prayer to myself ... we chatted, and when the tea was over ... "I can't believe it," she said, "the toothache is gone!"'

## Hope and Reassurance

I asked those I interviewed do they offer hope and reassurance to the people who come for their cure. The response was mixed; some people with cures will reassure and give hope, but most simply make their cure and are wary of offering false hope. Dr Patrick Logan believed firmly in the power of reassurance to aid healing. He wrote that 'the best medicine is reassurance and the ability to reassure a patient does not always go with a medical degree ... Folk curers ... have not forgotten that they are treating people and therefore they continue to practice successfully because they bring reassurance.'

A seventh son with a ringworm cure thought that 'you can reassure a person ... that they are going to be fine, and that's all they need to be told in order for them to be that ... people are their own best healers.' However, the man with a cure for blood pressure explained, 'I just tell them I've the cure made and hopefully it will be a good help to them.' An older woman who made a shingles cure had a strong belief in it, but she said, 'I will not guarantee it.' She knew that in some cases the condition cleared and the pain lingered.

## Different or Special

I also asked my interviewees do people see you as different or special. Generally, it was felt that within their communities they are not viewed as special, but the help they give to others is respected and acknowledged, via thanks, gifts and money. The majority of those with cures do not consider themselves to be different in any way.

A man with a popular skin cancer cure did not think he was special; '[I'm] just a farmer, that's all I am.' Another man who had been given three cures (shingles, ringworm and erysipelas) twenty years before I spoke to him reflected and said, 'I don't think that it made any difference after I got them.' A well-known healer acknowledged that some people see her as special because 'I have a gift', but 'I don't think of myself as special … I'm just an ordinary woman, with an ordinary life … and ups and downs like everybody else.'

## Seventh Daughters and Sons are Special

It is my belief that seventh daughters and sons are special; they are a unique and important part of the Irish healing tradition. I think others are of this opinion too. An elderly seventh daughter, who cured ringworm and other skin ailments, said that she had always been viewed as special, in particular when she was growing up, 'very special … very well-known … I was different to all my other sisters'. A younger seventh daughter remembered that when she was a child a number of people thought she was special. They would say to her, 'you were shined upon … you're God's gift!'

## Generosity

Generosity is a striking aspect of the cure tradition of Ireland. I found that people with cures are extremely generous with their time and energy, and in their willingness to help others, to ease them of their pain and problems.

There was an elderly man in east Sligo with two cures, for the head and the heart. He was friendly and sociable, and was never inconvenienced by the people coming to his home for them. 'I wouldn't have asked ... for it, unless I was willing to help ... and cure people.' He said that as a consequence of his heart cure there was always lots of oatmeal (an essential part of the cure) left over. 'I do feed it out to the birds in wintertime.' And the woman with a bleeding cure told me that whenever she came upon an accident or even heard of one, she said her special prayer. 'If we see or hear of an accident ... if you passed something on the road ... you'd hope you could do some good.'

# CHAPTER 13

# Faith, Success, Source and Passing on Cures

## Faith

**D**O PEOPLE HAVE TO BELIEVE in your cure for it to work, do they have to have faith in the cure? This was a question I always asked those I interviewed and the answer was overwhelmingly yes. I clarified 'faith' as meaning faith in the cure, rather than religious faith; for some people these two faiths are entwined. Those who seek a cure generally have faith in it and believe it will work, and this conviction is seen as contributing to the success of the cure.

Lenihan wrote of the people who sought help from wise woman Biddy Early: 'By coming to her first the suppliant displayed faith in her power, and it was this faith more than anything else that guaranteed the cure ... the very act of coming was a step nearer peace of mind.' Buckley had a very good understanding of the traditional cures and he thought that, 'To be cured, one must suspend critical judgement, rationality and common sense, and "believe" that one will recover. To some, this is merely an exercise in positive thinking: to others it is placing oneself in the hands of a merciful God.'

A seventh son thought that 'if a person comes ... looking for a cure, they wouldn't do it unless some part of them believed it could happen'.

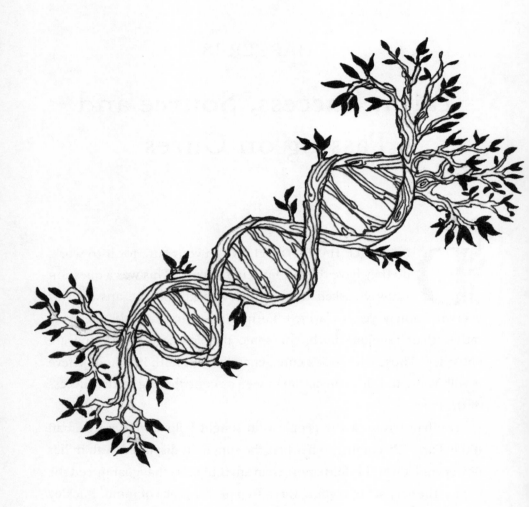

*A man who had a herbal cure for gallstones was given it by his mother;*
*he intended to pass it on to his daughter. Lots of cures are passed within*
*families from one generation to the next.*

Someone who had a cure for severe hoarseness explained, 'I do say ... don't come if you have no faith, it's a waste of time ... you won't be cured ... They have to think positive ... It's positive thinking really.' The man with a Bell's palsy cure also felt strongly that the person getting his cure must have faith in it. 'People have to have the belief in what they're coming for ... It's not something you try ... [it's something] you believe.'

## Faith Not Necessary

A small number of my interviewees felt that faith in their cure was not necessary (by those receiving it) for it to be effective. The majority of these people had herbal cures, like the man with a gallstones cure who told me that because his cure was primarily made from herbs, people did not have to believe in it for it to work; however, he said, 'It helps to think positive!'

Some with non-herbal cures also thought that the person did not have to believe in the cure for it to be successful, such as one man with a thrush cure. He normally helped babies and felt that even if the parents did not have faith in his cure, it would still work, as the child was separate to them. And a healer said that the majority of those who came to her believed she could heal. Now and then teenagers with skin problems were brought by their parents and the young person may have had no faith in the cure, but she recalled, they 'can be the very one that's healed'.

## Children's Faith

A few of the people I interviewed told me that their cure works very well for children. This may be because children are too young to doubt a cure and they can unquestioningly accept things which adults find hard to believe; they hold no negative thoughts about the cure. One of the faith healers I spoke to was aware that he had the most success 'with children under the age of four, who would have no belief in a God ... but yet ... they don't deny themselves the right to recover ... by being sceptical or doubtful'. Also, a man who made a sprain cure had found that 'if you're a sceptic it doesn't seem to work as well ... children especially and people who seem to be religious ... it works straight away'.

## Belief in Their Cure

Those who make cures invariably have a strong belief in their cure. One person who prepared an ointment for a burn said simply, 'I wouldn't make it, if I hadn't faith in it.' I met a woman who had been making her family strain cure for less than a year, but had great faith in it. Initially she was unsure as to how good it would be; 'the first three or four people that I did the cure for and it did work, I was totally gobsmacked!' A man with a cure for mumps put it logically; 'you wouldn't make it if you didn't believe in it' and 'they wouldn't come if they didn't believe in it'. He felt 'belief' was central to the healing process and that 'you can cure yourself with your mind, if you have ... belief'.

## Success

People with traditional cures believe them to be effective, to work most of the time. Many of my interviewees felt that because their cure had survived, because people kept coming for it and recommending it to others, then it must be successful. I think there is truth in this deduction. I also believe that an awareness of past successes of a cure most likely offers a degree of reassurance and hope to the person receiving it. This awareness is created by those who recommend the cure; who have found it to be helpful personally or who know of someone who has benefitted from it. In addition, those with cures may refer to their success rate when they are initially contacted or subsequently visited. Therefore, an expectation that the cure will work can exist prior to its administration, a positive expectation which is conducive to healing.

I did not attempt to look at the other side of the exchange, to speak to the people availing of cures and to hear their experiences. I have left this for someone else to investigate. I accepted in good faith the responses I got from those making cures with regard to their success rates. For example, the woman with a whooping cough cure told me that it had an 'excellent' success rate. She said that parents could be very anxious, 'so worried about their child ... they can't believe it after a week, that it is gone'.

An elderly woman who made an eczema cure thought that because it was popular this implied that it was effective. I had heard of this woman's cure through a former classmate, a nurse. She had tried everything to cure her young son's chronic eczema, to no avail. She became aware of the cure and decided to try it. To her surprise and delight the child was completely cured within three weeks. However, a friend used this ointment too on her little boy and found it to have minimal effect. As with most cures the success rate would appear to vary from person to person.

An elderly man believed that both his cures (for heart issues and headaches) were very effective. He had helped a variety of serious heart problems; 'people have told me ... they were due to go back to hospital for by-passes ... when they went back, they couldn't believe it ... they were in the clear ... and the doctor said, what happened here?' A healer, best known for helping skin problems, was realistic about the impact of her work. 'I say, now this should help, but not everybody is cured.' She recalled when a local radio station interviewed her and then carried out an informal survey of her cures, they found that her success rate was 'about 80 per cent'.

## Worse Before Better

It is believed that the condition can sometimes get worse, following the commencement of the cure, before it starts to get better; this is what I was told by a few of my interviewees. One woman's shingles cure was made over three consecutive days. She explained that after the first visit people often felt quite unwell and they told her 'it was very sore last night'. She believed this was a sign that the cure was working. The man with a hiatus hernia cure knew that one cure (three visits to him) was sufficient for most people. He too thought that the person could feel more unwell when they started the cure and he reassured them by saying, 'You have to get worse before you get better!'

## Cannot Cure Family

Some of those I interviewed told me that they are able to cure lots of people, but not members of their own family. This is an anomaly in the healing tradition of Ireland and the reason for its existence is unclear. Examples include one woman's well-known cure for warts which she inherited from her father. He was unable to get rid of her warts and she could not cure her children of this affliction. When her daughter had a wart, she went to the local pharmacy and bought a conventional treatment. She said that the women working there were highly amused as they regularly sent people to her for the cure!

A seventh son with a ringworm cure knew that he could not contract this infection, but his family could and unfortunately, he was not able to help them. 'Any blood relation I can't cure, even my mother had it and some of my brothers ... and I couldn't cure them.'

Meda Ryan has written that Biddy Early was allegedly unable to heal herself: 'Her insight and power was such that though she was able to help others, she was unable to use this gift in matters which concerned herself.'

## Source

What is the source of the healing, what causes the cure to take place? The replies to this question varied. A number of those with herbal preparations believed that the key to the cure was the plants they used; but the most common response was God. A woman who had a faith cure for bleeding told me it was 'the prayer, definitely ... without the prayer there is no cure ... a prayer is always heard'. Another woman believed her asthma cure was a combination of herself and God; 'inside me ... and the man above ... there is a power from him'.

Some people had a less clearly defined or broader understanding of what caused their cure to take place, like one of the seventh sons I met, who thought that the source of the healing was 'pure energy ... love and this pure form of energy are one and the same thing ... It's an energy that doesn't know defeat and doesn't know limitations.' A woman with a whooping cough cure said, 'I know I have a kind of a healing power ... I think most people have, if they want to delve into it.'

I contacted a seventh son living in Australia. He grew up in my local village and as a child cured many people of ringworm, including me. This man, now in his thirties, had lived abroad for years and rarely made his cure, but whenever he did, it was for an Irish person. He said, 'It seems to be only Irish people who have heard of these cures or believe in them.' As an adult and atheist reflecting on his cure from a distance, he said, 'I now believe that a lot of ailments can be cured by one's belief that you can beat something and recover from it. It is to this "Positive mental attitude" that I attribute a lot of the ability to "Cure" somebody.'

## Motivation for Making Cures

I asked my interviewees why do you make your cure? You have a choice, you could stop. I also asked them what effect (positive or negative) the cure had had on them, on their lives. The answers to these two questions often overlapped. A farmer with an eye cure said, 'It was handed down to me. I'd like to continue it.' He believed he would lose his cure if he stopped making it. Like most people with traditional cures, he did not think very often about his cure or try to analyse it. 'Those types of things, I wouldn't question too much … if they [the cures] work, they work.'

Someone who had a jaundice cure for many years reflected, 'I think we are here to help … that's what Christianity is supposed to be about.' Likewise, a woman with a migraine cure thought, 'If you're able to help somebody, why not … that's what life is all about … We're only passing through.' And a man who had a gallstones cure felt that 'If you do good for people … hopefully it will come around in some other form for you.'

## Sentimental Attachment

Many people had a strong sentimental attachment to their cure, especially if they had inherited it from a parent; this motivated them to keep making it. One woman was given a wart cure by her father. When he was dying in hospital, 'He just looked at me and says, I'm giving you the cure of warts.' She was reluctant to accept it and asked him, 'How am I supposed to do it?' He answered, 'You'll know yourself, all you do is touch them.' She lived in the original family home and worked next door in the veterinary clinic where her father had practised. She felt this element of continuity was one of the reasons he gave the cure to her, rather than another family member. Each time she made the cure, she thought of her father.

## Negative Affect

Cures can be accompanied by challenges for those who have them. Making a cure involves a commitment of energy and positivity, and particularly of time. People with cures have to fit them into their lives, to ensure that the cure is a workable part of their routine. Many have to be at home when the cure is collected or administered in person, they have to talk to strangers on the telephone and to welcome them into their house; these are aspects of the cure which some people find difficult and for which there is no (or little) tangible reward.

Two evenings per week people came to one woman's house to receive her strain cure. She had found it challenging to always be at home these two nights. 'I work five days a week ... it really is a commitment ... If you don't keep it to the days, it'll absolutely take over your life.' Another woman was well-known for her foot rot and back pain cures. She remembered people making appointments to come for a cure, and 'they wouldn't come at all and I could be waiting'.

A seventh son recalled that when he was a child (in the 1970s) he was consistently making his ringworm cure, 'every Monday and Thursday there was a queue ... my mother nearly used to have to give them tickets!' He wanted to be outside playing football with the other children, but instead he had to stay inside and cure people. In addition, his brothers would get annoyed with him because when a person came for the cure, they had to leave the sitting room (where the cure was made) and stop watching television!

## Cures and Poor Health

A handful of the people I interviewed mentioned an old belief; if you make a cure and help others, your own health will suffer. Lady Gregory gathered folklore at the beginning of the twentieth century in the west of Ireland and she recorded that priests who heal 'must lose something when they do cures – either their health or something else'. Anthony Buckley was told by an Ulster woman, who had a sprain cure and also poor personal health, that she wondered was the latter because she had the cure? 'She had heard that those who have the cure take upon themselves the sufferings of those they help.'

A man with a hernia cure said that he felt unwell after making it; 'funny enough ... I do suffer meself ... when I do the cure ... I do often find meself getting affected by it ... Maybe you do have to suffer with cures?' Similarly, the man whose cure was for Bell's palsy told me that now and then when he laid his hands on a trapped nerve, he felt heat. And that when the person had left, he could 'experience that [their] pain ... in my leg, or my shoulder, or my arm ... It doesn't last for very long.' He explained that 'after you complete the cure ... you feel pretty drained ... like shortness of breath ... The power that you have has left you, for a short period of time.'

## Passing on Cures

Most people with cures are eager to pass them on, if they are able to do so. Usually, a lot of attention is given to the choice of successor, someone who would be interested in the cure, would want it and would care for it. Cures are often passed to a younger family member, a daughter, son, niece or nephew. It can also help the continuation of the cure if it remains local or in the same place, such as the family home. One woman's cure for whooping cough had survived and thrived in this way: 'my mother had me here and I'm here with my children'. She planned to pass on her cure, to 'keep it in the family' and preferably in the same house.

I spoke to a man who held a strong belief in the traditional cures. He acquired his burn cure as a child when he licked a mankeeper. When I spoke to him, he said that if he happened upon one of these little newts, he would encourage whoever he was with to do likewise. 'I've done it with three of my own kids ... we just came on it when we were working out on the farm ... I got the three of them to lick it ... and I always try to make them aware how important it is to have it.'

If they are content to keep making it, the majority of people hold on to their cure until they are elderly. This is why the popular perception of someone with a cure is of an old person. It does not necessarily mean that their cure will die with them, though that can happen. Occasionally, cures may not be passed on because the person with the cure becomes ill and dies before they have chosen a successor. This was the reason I was frequently given during the course of my research as to why cures no longer existed. In some instances, younger people can be hesitant to ask an ageing relative about the future of a cure. For example, in 2006 I looked for a woman in south Sligo who had a herbal cure for erysipelas; I had interviewed her in 1986. I found her godson who said that the cure had sadly died with her. She had become sick unexpectedly and her family were reluctant to ask her for the cure because they felt she might then think that they thought she was going to die, which she did.

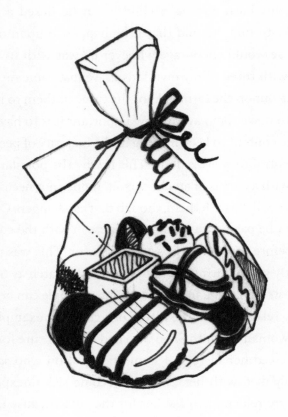

*Gifts, in thanks for cures, are common, and include flowers, chocolates, cakes, wine, whiskey, cards and groceries: tea, butter and potatoes.*

# CHAPTER 14

# Payment and Exchange, Modern Medicine and Cures

*※*

## Payment and Exchange

ITH REGARD TO GIVING SOMETHING in thanks or exchange for a cure, there are varying opinions. Those with cures generally have strong thoughts on the matter and they usually believe that their version of the tradition is the right one. An analysis of my research into this aspect is as follows; approximately two-thirds of the ninety-three people I interviewed accepted gifts in thanks for their cure, one-third did not accept money, and one-third accepted money. The situation was not clear-cut however, as the people who accepted money for their cure would equally take a gift and half of those who accepted money gave all or part of it to charity. A few individuals took absolutely nothing and a small number of people charged a fee for their cure or healing work.

I found that the tradition of exchange remains very strong; this is the belief that something, no matter how little, should be given in exchange for a cure. A gift is not asked for, but it is seen by many to be part of the cure process; it is an expression of thanks and an acknowledgement of the effort that the person with the cure has made. What is given can be small and inexpensive (often food or drinks), a prayer of gratitude would be welcomed or a simple thank you may suffice.

From her research in the latter half of the nineteenth century, Lady Wilde also noted that differing views existed concerning payment for cures. She wrote that, 'If a potion is made up of herbs it must be paid for in silver; but charms and incantations are never paid for, or they would lose their power. A present, however, may be accepted as an offering of gratitude.'

## Gifts

Most of my interviewees accepted and appreciated a gift in thanks for their cure. Gifts included flowers, chocolates, biscuits, cakes, sweets, beer, wine, whiskey, cigarettes, tobacco, mobile phone credit, gift vouchers, books, plants, perfume, socks, toys, holy pictures, thank you cards, Mass bouquet cards and groceries: tea, milk, sugar, butter and potatoes.

A seventh son with a cure for ringworm would not accept money for it, but he took gifts. When he was a child, a lot of groceries were given to his family; in later years people brought sweets to his children.

A farmer who had a mumps cure said, 'I was told that you should never take money for a cure', so people gave him chocolates, and the odd bottle of whiskey. In Meda Ryan's biography of Biddy Early, *The Wise Woman of Clare*, she writes that, 'Biddy preferred not to get money ... gifts in kind were more acceptable to her. This was in keeping with the old Irish tradition as it was believed that if the healer demanded payment, their powers would be taken away from them ... a jar of whiskey was a favourite present.'

## No Money

Many people with cures strongly believe that money should not be accepted for them, like the woman with a cure for warts who said, 'what I actually tell them is, if I take money or touch money it's not going to work'. If people insisted, she suggested they should donate to a local charity, but only at the end of the cure when the warts had disappeared. Likewise, a seventh daughter remembered that in childhood her mother had told her that 'she couldn't take money, that there'd be no cure in it if she took money out of their hand'.

## Accepting Money

Some people accept money for their cures, but I do not believe that they make money from them. Those receiving a cure are under no obligation to pay for it (unless there is a stated fee), and the amount they choose to give is discretionary. Cures often involve considerable time, energy and commitment from the people who make them; it is difficult to put a price on what they do.

One woman I met did not charge for her three cures, but she told me that she would take money to cover her costs, in particular for the eczema ointment she prepared. And an elderly man who had a bleeding cure said that most people phoned and asked him to make the cure, and he never heard from them again. Occasionally, they gave him money, and 'you won't offend people by refusing', or gifts, 'maybe a voucher for a meal'.

## Money to Charity

Many of the people who accept money for their cure do not keep it for personal use. It is common practice to give cure money to charity, such as the local hospice. A man who made a jaundice cure for years was seldom given a gift in thanks for it, as the written instructions which accompanied the herbal bottle stated that, 'No personal payment will be accepted in either cash or kind, but a donation to the Rehabilitation Centre would be greatly appreciated.' Another man with a cure for the eyes said, 'I don't charge ... If they feel like giving anything, give it to ... whatever charity they like.' If he was given money, he redirected it to a charitable organisation.

## Accepting Nothing

A few of the people I interviewed were adamant that they can accept nothing in return for their cure, like the man with a cure for shingles who informed me that he could not take anything, money, gifts or thanks. This was the way the cure was passed to him and he had adhered to the tradition for fifty years.

Nora Smyth came upon this belief too; she documented a County Down man who had three cures: 'He accepts no monetary offering otherwise the cure would not work, nor is the person supposed to thank him.' In addition, a teenage student in Armagh had warned her that, 'You should never say thank you to the person who is curing you as this might jeopardize the cure.'

Anthony Buckley recorded a prayer cure for bleeding in Northern Ireland, where the woman who had it would take nothing for it, not even thanks. She had told him that she asks the person looking for the cure to stand at her front door 'and after explaining the necessity of what she will do, she informs him that he will get better and slams the door. Where the patient has telephoned, she slams the phone down ... Thus she avoids hearing the fateful words "thank you"!'

## Charging a Fee

A handful of my interviewees had a modest set fee for their cures, usually if it was a herbal preparation. Some healers charged as well, but again the amounts were relatively small considering the time and attention they gave to each person. One man made a cure for gallstones with wild plants. He had a minimal price on his cure and he explained, 'there's some of the stuff I have to source myself. It's just to cover your own expenses.'

An elderly woman with a cure for gout charged a small amount of money. 'We had to put a charge on it, which we didn't like doing' but she remembered that they were inundated with gifts, chocolates, biscuits and whiskey; 'this place was like a shop!' Some of the money she received for her cure was given to charity.

## The Exchange Tradition

A seventh son, who healed ringworm, firmly believed that money must not be accepted for cures. However, he understood that a gift should be given in exchange for a cure. 'You weren't allowed to take money, but people did bring a gift and that was a very important thing ... There's an exchange.' Having said this, the gift could be little and simple: 'They could gather shells on the beach ... or make a small bread.' He felt that the thinking about and the offering of the gift was a significant aspect of the cure, as it allowed the person to play a role in the healing process.

One man made his sprain cure for four decades and he told me that 'you're not supposed to ask anything for it ... [but] they feel they must give something if the cure is to work ... I think this is probably the residue of the barter system.' Another man, with an eye cure, accepted gifts from those he helped and he also felt that this element of exchange was important. He was given it by an old woman and she thought 'that a cure wasn't fulfilled until something passed between'.

The woman who had been making a cure for sprains for half a century told me that the neighbour she inherited it from instructed her to 'exchange a coin'. Therefore, she only accepted a coin, not paper money, for her cure and this she passed on to either a charity or the Church. 'If they want to give me a coin ... I'd light a candle for them, I never made use of cure money ... I don't even put it in with me own money,' she said proudly.

## Modern Medicine and Cures

People with traditional cures have a lot of respect for modern medicine and they utilise its services. With regard to their cure, it varied as to whether people believed the doctor's medicine could be taken in tandem with the cure or if medication should stop once the cure started; most were in the former camp. Many of them asked the person looking for their cure if they had been to a doctor, what the diagnosis was, and what medicines they were taking.

## Continuing/Stopping Medication

The man with a Bell's palsy cure was aware that many of those who came for it had sought medical advice first. He believed that 'the charm isn't affected by ... any medicines ... They can go and take whatever tablets they want.' One healer sometimes advised people to visit their doctor if she thought they were seriously ill. She phoned them subsequently to check that they had done this. If their problem had a psychological dimension, she 'would advise them to see a counsellor'.

Some people believed that the doctor's medication had little effect on the problem their cure was for or that it would make it worse. For others, they felt it was best if medicine was not taken in conjunction with their cure and that the two approaches to healing should be kept separate. A woman who had a cure for shingles recommended that people did not take her cure and medication simultaneously; 'if they want to finish the tablets from the doctor and then start the herbal cure ... I advise them not to use them together.'

A man with a thrush cure told me that the child would normally have seen the family doctor before they came to him and he felt that the treatment given may have caused the condition to deteriorate. A seventh daughter said that plenty of the people who availed of her ringworm cure had tried modern medicine with no success. She believed that the recommended creams only spread the infection.

## Sympathetic Doctors

I learnt that some doctors and health professionals are sympathetic to and acknowledge the value of traditional cures. A German mountaineer told me that when he was living in south Leitrim in the late 1980s his son developed thrush. He took the little boy to the GP, who explained that his treatment would take three weeks to work, but that there was a local man with the cure and he could clear it in two days. So, he brought the child to this man, who breathed into the boy's mouth, and as predicted, after two days the infection had disappeared. In 2006 I interviewed a Sligo farmer who was well-known in his area for the cure of thrush. He was aware of a few doctors suggesting his cure to the parents of babies with this problem.

A seventh son with a ringworm cure lived adjacent to an urban medical centre and a GP there regularly sent patients to him. A seventh daughter in rural Mayo also cured ringworm and other skin ailments. Her local doctor encouraged many who had chronic skin conditions, especially children, to go to her. And a man in north Leitrim, who made a herbal cure for shingles, knew that most of the people who requested it had been diagnosed already by a doctor. Occasionally GPs had recommended his cure.

There was a woman in south Sligo who had a cure for warts. Now and then, the nearby family doctor advised patients with this affliction to visit her. In 2007 my friend went to a large, sophisticated pharmacy in Sligo town to buy a treatment for her child's warts. The young female assistant there showed her a variety of creams, but then discreetly told her that she would be better off taking the boy for the cure and proceeded to give her this woman's name.

A degree of overlap currently exists in Ireland between traditional cures and modern medicine; this is an interconnection which is little-known about and rarely discussed publicly. I found it thought-provoking to read social scientist Vincent Tucker's writings on health and healing. He argued that the dominant biomedical model of health in Western societies was reductionist as it overfocused on the biological, at the expense of other interrelated factors: social, economic, political, environmental and personal. He believed that this model excluded 'other ways of understanding and practising medicine', and he reminded us that all knowledge is partial, and reflective of its social and historical context. Ultimately, he advocated for 'the adoption of a more holistic or ecological approach to health ... Patients should be free to seek the knowledge and help most appropriate to their health needs ... the holistic approach is more multi-dimensional, taking into account the energy system, the realm of consciousness, the spiritual dimension, the interpersonal and the social dimension.'

## Charms and Quacks

When investigating the traditional cures, I came across the terms charm (the cure) and quack (the person with the cure). There was not widespread usage of these words; the expression charm appears to be most common in the province of Ulster/Northern Ireland. A man who lived in County Armagh made a cure for Bell's palsy. He referred to it as the charm rather than cure, which he felt was a very strong word. A woman from Monaghan had a shingles cure and she said that when people were sick, they looked for the cure and then they came for it, or as she put it, 'they come for the charm'. And in Tyrone, a farmer with a cure for heart fever told me that if people were in need, 'you don't turn your back on that, if you've got the charm of the cure'.

Henry Glassie wrote about the folklore and history of an Ulster community in the early 1980s, and he alluded to cures which 'usually combine herbal concoctions with prescribed procedures, subtle prohibitions, and a "charm" in which the real power lies'. He elaborated by saying, 'The cure is administered with a "charm", a prayer, a reciprocating expression of gratitude to God.'

In the folk medicine research Professor Michael Doherty carried out via veterinary surgeons (1999–2000), he also encountered the word charm in Ulster. With regard to the bleeding cure, feedback from vets in County Antrim reported that, 'The person with the charm requires to know the sex of the animal and its colour' and that, 'A progressive pedigree beef breeder always calls the "charmer" to resolve any bleeding problems.' This study found that faith cures for bleeding were equally utilised by Protestants and Catholics in contemporary Northern Ireland.

Nora Smyth recalled the fascinating history associated with a particular County Down cure. Many years ago, an old woman lay dying; she was unsure of who to pass her charms to and, 'Fearing that perhaps these might fall into the wrong hands and be used for monetary advantage, she got up out of her sick bed, went down to the bog near her house and consigned the nine charms to the bog.' So, the man who subsequently got her cures had to literally go into the bog each time one was needed, and reclaim the charm!

In the interview I conducted with a seventh daughter who cured warts as well as ringworm, her mother joined us. This woman lived in rural Longford and she mentioned the term 'quack doctor' a number of times when referring to people with cures. For example, she said, 'It's seldom a doctor will recommend a quack doctor.' She was remembering a friend who had shingles some years previously and who was told by his GP to get the cure.

The dictionary definition of a quack is 'an unqualified person who claims medical knowledge or other skills ... a quack doctor'. The terms quack or quack doctor were expressions I came upon infrequently. When speaking to a north Sligo man who had a cure for severe hoarseness, he said that people usually go to a doctor before a cure; 'If that doesn't work, then they look for a quack.' Another man, in Donegal, told me that sometimes he had gone to a hospital and made his shingles cure for a patient there. However, he was reluctant to do this as he felt doctors and nurses were not supportive of the old cures, and they called people like him quacks.

Psychiatric nurse and lecturer Peter Nolan documented some traditional cures in north Roscommon in 1988. He called those with cures folk healers or quacks, and he believed that, 'In Ireland "quack" is not a derogatory title. It simply refers to someone not medically trained but who is regarded as having "the cure."' He concluded that, 'The quacks are held in high regard ... I spoke to caring people who live in caring communities.'

# CHAPTER 15

# Healing Threads, Clays, Cloths and Stones

A S WELL AS SEEKING CURES from particular individuals, some Irish people use physical items for healing and protection; these include straining threads, holy clays, St Brigid cloths and curing stones. I investigated a number of objects, locations and beliefs which are part of these traditional approaches to good health.

## Straining Threads

A straining thread is an ordinary piece of thread or wool which becomes an essential component of some cures for strains and sprains; it is tied around the damaged area. People call this type of injury either of the two names and the terms would appear to be interchangeable; I think strain is an older, more traditional phrase. The use of these healing threads is not uncommon. A young woman from north Leitrim informed me that following a bad foot sprain in 2003, she got the cure locally. She went to the regional hospital as well, and when the orthopaedic doctor there

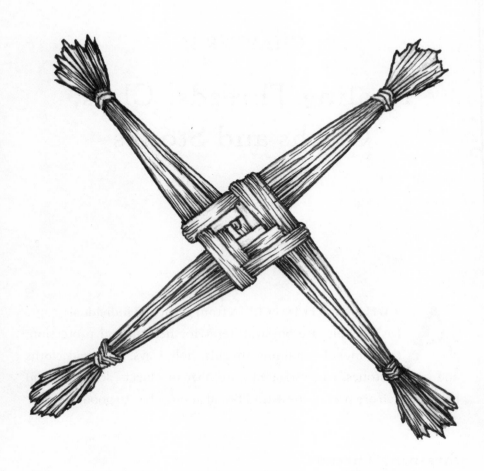

*Brigid was a pre-Christian fertility goddess and a Christian saint; her cross, made of rushes, is also a sun symbol.*

saw the straining thread wrapped around her ankle he was amused and said that he often had Leitrim people in his clinic with these threads.

In a small, peaceful burial ground in east Sligo there is a straining thread cure. Seven big, smooth, round stones, with a rectangular upright stone in the middle of them, lie on a large stone slab. To cure a strain a length of wool must be wound around the upright stone. Each of the round stones are then turned over, preferably using one hand, and moving in a clockwise direction as prayers are recited. An elderly, local man told me that five Hail Marys, five Our Fathers and five Glory Bes should be said. A different thread, left by a previous person, is removed from the upright stone and tied around the sprain. The ritual is called 'lifting the thread'. A prayer is said too for the saint (possibly Aireidh) who placed the cure there, hundreds of years ago, having first used it on his lame horse. The cure can be made on behalf of the injured individual and the piece of wool given to them. The straining thread should be allowed to fall off naturally and this is believed to occur when the strain is healed. This cure has remained popular into the twenty-first century for humans and animals.

I interviewed a middle-aged man in rural Sligo who had cures for headaches, the heart and strains. The latter was his most popular cure; some weeks he 'could have three or four people'. He frequently helped animals with this cure, especially cattle and horses. To make it, he took three pieces of white thread, 'ordinary sewing thread', and holding them together he made nine knots at regular intervals along the threads. He said three blessings while he was performing this ritual. The length of the thread depended on the injury, as it could be for a strained wrist or a waist.

In private, after the thread had been collected, he prayed for the injured person using their name; if the cure was for an animal, he incorporated the name of the owner. He had memorised the (secret) prayers and it took ten to fifteen minutes to complete them. People were told not to remove the thread; 'the cure isn't finished until the thread falls off'. He thought that his cure was connected to the straining thread in the old cemetery, and when he said the prayers for the cure, he always acknowledged the saint of this burial ground. He felt that some of the power (the source) of the cure was coming from this saint and that his own role was minor. 'I'm only just an instrument' was how he explained it.

I also spoke to a young man (early twenties) who made a sprain cure. He lived at the edge of a large town in the north-west, and worked on his family's farm and in a factory. He started making the cure as a teenager and had inherited it from his grandmother, with whom he was very close. Initially, he did a few things to the white cotton thread, which he kept secret. He then gave this thread to the person with the injury, and directed them to tie it on over the sprain using three knots and to say a blessing. The three knots had to be tied one on top of the other, and as the first knot was tied he said, 'In the name of the Father', with the second he said 'Son', and 'Holy Spirit' accompanied the third knot.

He too stressed the importance of letting the thread fall off in its own time, and believed that if it was more than a sprain the thread could remain there for weeks or even months. Usually, people did not come to see him in person; rather, he made the cure, left the thread in an envelope with the instructions at his family home and it was collected. He worked abroad for some time, and when people came looking for the cure he was contacted and posted it to them, or 'when I went to England ... I always used to make up a few and leave them at home for me mother ... so she'd just hand them out.'

In Donegal there was a woman with an asthma cure and a lesser-known one for sprain. She had used it to help family members and animals (horses, cows and bulls), and she told me that 'it has all worked'. A string, which is 'the cord that comes out of the potato bag' was central to her cure. The length of the string varied. 'I always do it bigger for horses.' She ran the cord up and down between the thumb and index finger of both her hands, saying prayers as she did this; she mentioned 'the name of the person ... or the animal' and the injury they had. She then blessed the string three times with holy water, and 'you tie a knot in it ... and tie it on the person ... the knot has to stay to the front'. If people could not come to her, or if it was for an animal, she posted the cord to them. Unlike many other straining threads, this woman told people to remove the string when they felt healed.

## Holy Clays

The following are a selection of clays from locations around Ireland that are believed to have healing and protective properties; currently, they are all well utilised by the public. These special clays are often associated with priests and saints, and in particular, with the graves of certain holy men and women.

The final resting place of Fr Magauran (d. 1837) is among the ruins of a sixteenth-century abbey near the small town of Dromahair in north Leitrim. People take clay from his grave and have great belief in its curative ability. However, the clay must be returned once it has served its purpose. I stopped at the abbey in 2004 and I found a soggy, little note at his burial site which read, 'Mary, this is the clay that was taken off the priest's grave. Hold it for a week or two. Say a prayer each day for a cure for your foot, and when Bob is coming up again, you can send it up with him. We'll get it back on the grave, Paula.'

I revisited this old monastic settlement two years later and I spoke to a man who lived close by. He told me that this clay was used to help a variety of ailments. People contacted him from every part of Ireland, from England and the USA, requesting the clay. He forwarded it and instructed them to keep it close (in their pocket or handbag, or under their pillow) for nine days, to say prayers for a cure every day and then to post it back to him. The specified prayers were five Our Fathers, Hail Marys and Glory Bes, and one Creed; three prayers should be said too for Fr Magauran, one Our Father, Hail Mary and Glory Be. A corner of the concrete slab which covered the grave had been cut out to allow easy access to this healing clay. Lots of the people who came in search of a cure here had left small personal items: keyrings, cutlery, coins, toys, shells, flowers, rosary beads and cigarettes.

I interviewed an elderly woman who lived on a small farm in east Sligo; she made a cure for whooping cough which was connected to Fr Magauran. She had a giant scapular consisting of two padded fabric squares, joined by two long, narrow strips of material, with a large gap in between. The sick child had to be put through the gap three times as a blessing was said. She explained that it was 'a religious cure' which was given to her great-grandmother by Fr Magauran in the early nineteenth century. It had been passed down through the generations of her family and the women members had taken good care of it. She felt it was 'very precious'.

In the past scapulars were part of the habit of Roman Catholic clergy. A man with an eye cure remembered his mother telling him that in the penal times (eighteenth century) if a priest celebrated Mass secretly in a house, he left a cure in that home. The Catholic Church in Ireland grew steadily in power and influence during the late 1800s/early 1900s, and it dominated Irish life for most of the twentieth century. Many people felt that priests had healing abilities. Cambridge (UK) academic Richard Breen conducted folklore research in rural Kerry in the 1970s and he found that a belief in 'priestly power' continued to exist there. He wrote that priests were thought to have supernatural powers which 'took two opposing forms – of cursing those who went against him or broke the laws of the Church ... and curing'.

Daingean is a little town in County Offaly (the central lowlands) through which the sleepy Grand Canal flows; yet it is just 10 km south of the M6 motorway. In an old cemetery near the town, you will find the grave of Fr Mullen; Andrew Mullen was born locally in 1790 and when he died twenty-eight years later in north Carlow, this priest had developed a healing reputation. The story goes that the people of Daingean wanted their native son returned, so five weeks after his death they dug up his body only to find that it had not decomposed (a sign of his closeness to God), and they brought it to its current resting site.

A very large, rectangular stone slab covers the grave, but it is elevated 30 cm from the ground on four plinths. This means that those looking for cures can easily remove the clay and some lie on the earth under the tombstone. A lot of people come to Fr Mullen's place of burial to pray, to request help with whatever worries or illnesses they have, or simply to find peace and quiet. Those who visit tend to leave something behind; the big, white crucifix and the brick-roofed 'shrine' at the head of this special grave were adorned with fresh flowers, plants, lanterns, coins, holy statues, scapulars, numerous rosary beads, a hurley stick and a boxing medal. An unofficial 'pilgrimage' to this grave takes place on Good Friday (Easter) and is well attended by people from all over the country.

Inis Oírr, in Galway Bay, is the smallest and most easterly of the three low, stony Aran Islands. Just 8 km of Atlantic Ocean separate it from north Clare, and today lots of tourists take this boat journey and temporarily expand the island's population of 280 people. Leaba Chaomháin (bed of Caomhán) is the grave of the patron saint of this Irish-speaking island, and it is located in the cemetery close to the pier and village. I was interested in the burial site of this holy man as I had read that in years gone by islanders in need of a cure lay on his grave, and that during storms they took sand from the grave and cast 'it upon the troubled waters to pacify the sea and bring the fishermen safe to shore'.

This information was in *Island Funeral*, a book of beautiful, colourful and dramatic photographs taken by Bill Doyle when he visited Inis Oírr in June 1965. His arrival on the island coincided with the funeral of an elderly man, *an scéalaí* (the storyteller), and the photos he took of the coffin being carried across the white strand under an azure sky could have been taken a hundred years earlier; men in homespun tweed trousers, waistcoats and caps, wearing handmade cowhide shoes, and women in black shawls and scarlet petticoats.

I visited Inis Oírr in 2017, fifty-two years after Doyle, and found that the graveyard, a hill of sand above the rocky shoreline, had changed little. At the centre of it is Teampall Chaomháin, a tenth-century sunken and roofless stone church, which is in constant danger of being engulfed by sand. The saint is buried beside his chapel, and because his grave is also sunken below the more recent headstones and is threatened by blowing sands, it is now covered by a little, stone 'house'. Five steps descend to the oak door of the tomb, passing a *ballán* stone which has a circular depression cut into it, a water font. Inside the confined space the grave slab lies about one metre below, it has a 'pillow' stone, and is inscribed with a large, intricate crucifix and Christ figure. Caomhán's 'bed' was clean and tidy, with a simple 'altar' above it, a few candles, plastic flowers and photographs of a teenage boy.

I talked to a man (in his early sixties) tending his father's grave nearby, in preparation for Mass in the burial ground a few days later on 14 June, the feast day (*pátrún*) of St Caomhán. He told me that fishermen used to take sand from the saint's grave with them when they went to sea in their small *curacha* (canvas-covered rowing boats), that the bigger *húicéirí* boats used to lower their sails as a sign of respect to the saint when they passed, and that some people still go to Caomhán's 'bed' to ask for help and healing.

St Mogue's clay comes from an island in a little lake near Bawnboy in north Cavan, not far from the border with Northern Ireland. Legend says that Mogue (or Maedoc), an early Christian saint and missionary, was born on this island c.555. The special clay is taken from within the walls of the church the saint founded there. His clay is understood to have protective properties. Patrick Logan wrote that the clay from St Mogue's Island 'was kept in the house to protect it against high winds or, if carried by a traveller, it protected him against disease or injury during his journey'. He was aware of a Cavan woman who had a son flying with the RAF in the Second World War; she had sent him the clay 'which he carried with him and his planes always came home safely'.

On the day I went to find this holy clay, while standing on the shore gazing across to the island, I met a helpful local couple. They gave me some of the clay, information about it and a cup of tea. The clay is dark brown and fine, with bits of root through it. Many people who live in the vicinity, as well as those from farther afield, keep small amounts of the clay in their cars and tractors. It is believed to prevent accidents and to protect against fire, so people have it in their homes too. In addition, the clay is thought to offer protection from drowning, and I was told of a woman who was a passenger on the ill-fated *Titanic* in 1912; she survived because she had the clay in her possession. Today, as part of the annual community festival (held in early August), boat trips to St Mogue's Island take place, along with a 'blessing of the graves' there and lakeside refreshments.

In the hills of north-west Donegal, close to the majestic Glenveagh National Park, there lived a middle-aged man who was a farmer and part-time builder. He and his family were the custodians of Gartan clay, a fine, white clay that was believed to have protective qualities. In the past, the person carrying it was felt to be protected from lightning, drowning and fire. When I visited, people used it for general personal protection and to assist them with any problems they had. It was also used to help cure health concerns like cancer, bad backs and arthritis.

'If you've that belief [in the clay], you can use it to help whatever ails you,' he explained.

Donegal people are particularly attached to Gartan clay; many keep it in their cars, especially young people and some professional rally drivers. Fishermen and those who sail take this clay with them to sea. He recalled two young men who had recently attempted to row across the Atlantic, but capsized. Luckily, a Glenties man had sent them this protective clay before they set out on their adventure and they were rescued. He knew of someone who had survived the 2004 Indian Ocean tsunami; they too had the clay with them. The most famous story connected to Gartan clay is that of a local woman who was due to travel on the *Titanic*; on the day of departure, she realised that she had forgotten the clay so she went home to get it, thereby missing her train and ultimately the doomed ship.

The farmer's hospitable wife was very involved with this clay as well; she helped him prepare it and gave it out to the numerous people who came looking for it. Together they formed the clay into small discs (thumbnail size, 1 cm deep), by mixing it with holy water, cut out the rounds, imprinted a cross on top of each one and left them to dry. There was no charge for the clay and everyone who wanted it was given a small portion. All ages and all types of people got Gartan clay; they came from every corner of Ireland, most notably Northern Ireland, and from England, America, Australia and New Zealand. Once a year a bus full of Queen's University Belfast students and their lecturers arrived, and they were each given a disc of clay.

The tradition surrounding Gartan clay was that only the male members of his family could move it from its secret location. He referred to this task as 'lifting the clay' and he did it twice a year. This was the way in which the clay has been 'handed down from generation to generation'. Both he and his wife were anxious that their sons kept the tradition going, so he had already shown them where and how to lift the clay, and what prayers to say. He was unsure as to the history of Gartan clay and its link to his family, but he knew that it was associated with Colmcille (St Columba) who was born nearby.

I made enquiries locally regarding the origins of Gartan clay and was told this story; Eithne, a noblewoman and mother of Colmcille, had just given birth to him (AD 521) when she had to flee attackers. She left a trail of blood behind which this man's ancestors covered up with clay, and in thanks for saving her and her baby, Eithne gifted them this holy clay. I was also informed that many Donegal men fighting in the trenches of the First World War had taken Gartan clay with them for protection.

Close by is the carved stone high cross erected by Lady Adair of Glenveagh Castle in 1911 to mark the reputed birthplace of the saint. Beside the cross are the ruins of a megalithic tomb, as well as a large, flat slab of stone, indented with small holes and littered with coins. It was on this rock, known as Leac na Cumha (flagstone of homesickness or parting sorrow), that Eithne gave birth to Colmcille. The saint is thought to have lain here before he departed for Iona in Scotland, to have blessed this stone and to have left a cure there. Those wanting a cure for loneliness or grief lie on it, and over the years many reluctant Donegal emigrants used it before they started their journey to foreign shores. The setting is pastoral and peaceful, and I can see how people would find solace there.

As I was conducting my fieldwork a number of people spoke to me of Tory clay, which has a reputation for keeping rats at bay. So, in August of 2007, I made the choppy crossing to this remote island, 12 km off the north Donegal coast. Toraigh (Tory) has about 140 inhabitants, its own style of painting and a king! Irish is the native tongue of the islanders. The special clay can be found close to An Baile Thiar (west town) where there is a ruined, early Christian oratory, Móirsheisear (church of the seven). Remembered in folklore are the seven people, strangers, who were laid to rest here (six men and one woman) having drowned nearby when their boat foundered.

The woman was buried outside the little church in a small, enclosed area known as Uaigh na Mná Rialta (grave of the nun). It is from this 'grave' that the protective clay is 'lifted' and this can only be done by the eldest member of a particular family on the island. I called to their door, and was told that there are no rats on Tory and that the clay is still popular, especially with fishermen. It had been used for decades by Donegal people, their relatives and friends, to drive rats out of houses, barns and boats, and to prevent them entering.

Dorothy Harrison Therman published her *Stories from Tory Island* in 1989 and she noted that this clay was used as well 'to protect fishermen from the dangers of the sea ... [from] whales and basking sharks... Dónal assured me that it was good for all kinds of travel, or anything that meant harm to me.'

## Brigid's Cloths

Brigid is the most important female saint in Ireland (second only to Patrick), and her feast day is 1 February, the first day of spring. But Brigid was also a pre-Christian fertility goddess, revered in many cultures throughout Europe, and associated with healing, poetry and fire; her name means 'fiery arrow'. Folktales recount that Brigid's father was the Dagda, the Tuatha Dé Danann father god, who dwelt at Newgrange (the great passage tomb). Mary Condren believes that, 'Upon its arrival in Ireland, Christianity had to reckon, not only with the warriors, but also with the most powerful female religious figure in all of Irish history: Brigit ... a folk image whose shadows still move over Ireland.'

Anne O'Dowd has written that, 'Brigid the goddess had a relatively easy transition from paganism to Christianity, and to her role as St Brigid.' She cites a sixth-century directive issued by the Pope to the

Bishop of Canterbury, urging 'Christian missionaries not to destroy pagan places of worship but to bless them and transform them into Christian places of worship.'

Robert Graves recalled that in Roman times there was a strong devotion to Brigit across Britain, in particular by naming sacred wells after her (Bridewell). He documented a Cornish cure for scalds, which he understood was an 'invocation to the local Brigit Triad':

> Three Ladies came from the East,
> One with fire and two with frost,
> Out with thee, fire, and in with thee, frost.

The instructions for this cure were that, 'One dips nine bramble leaves in spring water and then applies to the scald; the charm must be said three times to each leaf to be effective.'

Today in Ireland simple rush crosses (both sun and cross symbols) are made to mark the saint's feast day, especially by schoolchildren. These crosses are used as a form of blessing and protection for the homes (and stables) they will adorn. The crosses should be burned at the end of each winter and the freshly made ones put in their place, to herald the arrival of spring, abundant growth and new life.

The traditional belief is that St Brigid is out and about on the eve of her feast day, travelling across the land and blessing it. Therefore, on this night people place a cloth outside, known as *brat Bhríde* (Brigid's mantle or cloak), which they feel will subsequently possess healing properties. O'Dowd unearthed folklore collected in 1947 in Erris, north Mayo, describing the activities of St Brigid's Eve:

> A good fire was put down, the animals were bedded in clean
> straw and the family awaited Brigid's visit. The man of the
> house arranged the *Brat Bríde* (a garment to be imbued

with the saint's blessing to provide protection for all for the coming year), ate some of the meal and then asked the family to welcome Brigid into the home.

In 2006 I was teaching in a little country school in south Sligo. The children there told me that their families put outside blue and white cloths (usually a checked tea towel) on St Brigid's Eve, and that these cloths could be rubbed on any injured part of the body for the following year. One girl added that if the cloth was red and white it could cure throat problems. A woman from a small town in the same region said that she used her St Brigid's cloth particularly for headaches; she slept with it over her head if the pain was severe. O'Farrell noted that on St Brigid's Day 'people tied Saint Brigid's ribbon (*Ribín Bhríde*) to doorknobs; then they kept it to wind around the head to cure headaches'. A support worker for the Traveller community in a large town in the north-west informed me that some Traveller women put out a (white) cloth for St Brigid to bless the night before 1 February and that they then used it to ease the pain of childbirth.

Tradition says that St Brigid was born at Faughart, County Louth, in AD 453, close to the Northern Ireland border; the mighty, ancient tale of the bull raid (the *Táin*) was played out nearby. The true story of her life will never be known, but a strong narrative is that her mother was a slave, her father a chieftain and that she grew up in the house of a druid, working the farm and tending to the animals. In the various accounts of Brigid's life pagan and Christian elements are continuously interwoven. As a young woman she is thought to have converted to Christianity and to have established her famous monastery at Kildare (Cill Dara, church of the oak). Proinsias Mac Cana felt that 'no clear distinction can be made between the goddess and the saint and that in all probability Brighid's great monastery of Kildare was formerly a pagan sanctuary'. The thirteenth-century Church of Ireland cathedral at the centre of the town is named after St Brigid and it is believed to be on the site of her original church. There is a small community of Brigidine nuns still living in Kildare, keeping her flame alight.

An old graveyard is situated on the Hill of Faughart, just off the highway which has linked Ulster and the other provinces of Ireland for thousands of years. Its most famous incumbent is Edward Bruce, a Scot of noble birth, brother of Robert, and briefly the self-proclaimed King of Ireland; he was defeated by the English and died in the Battle of Faughart (1318). Within this tranquil burial ground is St Brigid's holy well, a short distance from her popular shrine further down the hillside. A stone hut has been built over the water source, which is sunken and accessed by a flight of broad steps. At the entrance to the little, dark well two long-handled, metal jugs hang, enabling people to collect water safely.

What I found interesting about this holy well was the number and diversity of personal belongings that have been left there. The sprawling laurel tree adjacent to it has been transformed into a colourful rag tree. It is weighed down with numerous items, apparently whatever people happened to have with them on the day they visited, which they have tied to this thriving tree. These included shoelaces, strings, tissues, hair bobbles, handkerchiefs, keyrings, measuring tapes, holy medals, photos of children, inhalers, cigarette lighters, plastic milk bottles, air fresheners, lots of socks and many, many scarves of every colour blowing in the wind. It is as if St Brigid gives us her cloths for healing and we leave our cloths in thanks for her help.

Brigid is associated with the protection and healing of animals. Professor Dáithí Ó hÓgáin wrote that, 'Brighid was a sort of guardian-goddess of domestic animals. This suggestion is strengthened by the cult of St Brighid, who is in folk culture the patroness of farm animals and whose feast day is the first day of spring. It was once known as Oímelg, meaning "lactation".' An east Leitrim farmer, with a cure for hiatus hernia, had a firm belief in St Brigid's ability to cure his animals. If his livestock were in trouble, he said a prayer to her to help them: 'I seen it happening with cows calving ... every time I go near me shed ... I do say a prayer to St Brigid.' His parents had huge faith in the saint too and there was a holy well close by dedicated to her.

In 2010 an elderly woman, who lived in south Leitrim and had a number of cures, told me of a cure to help an animal 'clean' (pass the placenta) after giving birth. It was connected to St Brigid whom she said 'was great with animals'. The night before her feast day, when 'she's supposed to come around', people left a large cloth sack outside, one that would be used for storing grain. The following morning, they brought it indoors and kept it safe. 'If you've a cow or a sheep that cannot clean ... put it around them on their back.' Tie the sack on and leave it there for a few days, and she assured me, 'you'll need no vet!' This was an old tradition in her area, but she knew that farmers still believed in it; 'there's people round here do it all the time'. O'Farrell recorded the custom of draping a *crios Bhríde* (Brigid's belt/girdle) made from hay or straw 'over the neck of a calving cow or on a fidgety milch cow to quieten her'.

## Healing Stones

St Dominic's Stone lies in the field which surrounds a handsome, sixteenth-century ruined abbey on the shore of Lough Arrow in south-east Sligo. This *ballán* stone is on a low hill beside a lone hawthorn tree and near the track leading to the old church. About 30 cm tall, it is placed on top of a rough boulder. A Christian monogram (a crucifix, bisecting the letters IHS) has been carved into the side of the stone facing the abbey. In the flat upper surface of the *ballán* there is a circular hole, 13 cm in diameter and 5 cm deep. The water which naturally lodges here is used as a wart cure; simply wash the warts with this water.

One meaning for the word *ballán* is 'a rock with a cup-shaped hole', and sometimes these eye-catching depressions are paired with a smooth, round stone which sits neatly in the hollow. Most likely of pre-Christian origin, these unusual stones can be found solo or in groups and at a variety of locations across Ireland. They are associated with healing and Dr Fleetwood noted that in particular they were supposed to be helpful to those with rheumatism and eye diseases. *Ballán* stones may also have had a functional use, such as for grinding corn.

Glendalough (valley of two lakes), deep in the Wicklow Mountains, is one of Ireland's biggest tourist destinations; over 600,000 people visit it annually. Despite its popularity, this wooded glen remains beautiful and peaceful, with a hint of wildness. St Kevin founded a monastic settlement here in the sixth century, and many of the buildings have survived the years, the weather and the Viking raids. There is an imposing gateway, a small cathedral, a little, stone-roofed church, an impressive round tower, an old cemetery and much more. In 2017 I went there in search of the Deer Stone, traditionally linked to cures and one of approximately thirty *ballán* stones that were to be found at Glendalough.

This curious stone rests on the verge of the pedestrian Green Road which leads from the visitor centre to the Upper Lake, beside a wooden footbridge and path into the monastic 'city'. It is part of a jumble of large boulders, possibly a collapsed megalithic tomb, that most of the modern-day 'pilgrims' (tourists) stroll past without giving a second glance. The Deer Stone is an excellent example of a *ballán*; a medium-sized stone, flat-topped, with a circular indentation (diameter 30 cm, tapering to a depth of 15 cm) cut into the middle of it.

I found no evidence of this stone being utilised for healing purposes when I visited, but the water that had collected in it looked to me like a classic cure for warts. Janet and Colin Bord investigated the Deer Stone in the 1980s, and they documented that it 'should be visited by the patient on Sunday, Tuesday and Thursday in the same week, and each time he or she must go round it seven times on bare knees'.

Legend says that St Kevin tried to help one of his workmen whose wife had died in childbirth. The saint commanded a wild doe to come to this stone every day and to allow herself be milked into the hollow. The deer's milk was then given to the baby, who survived, and hence the name of the stone. I was intrigued when I came across a reference by archaeological researcher Pádraig Meehan to the *cailleach* (the goddess) and her connection to deer; 'she milks deer as often as she milks cows; her wealth is the wealth of nature ... Whether depicted as a deer goddess, a corn goddess or as a deity governing winter, the core themes of the *Cailleach* in legend and folklore are decay, renewal and cyclical temporality.' It may be that the Deer Stone's source of abundance and healing is the pre-Christian goddess.

There is a 'well' dedicated to St Patrick in the woods of south Tyrone, not far from the town of Augher and the border with County Monaghan. A short trail leads through tall larch trees and lush, green ferns to Patrick's 'Chair'. It is a dramatic sight to come upon in the forest; a giant stone cut to create a simple throne on which two adults can comfortably sit. The information sign at the car park describes it as a 'druid stone' and tells the visitor that a wish made sitting there will come true, providing it is kept secret.

The path descends from the little ridge on which the 'chair' perches to a rag tree. This is a scrawny holly bush to which socks, ribbons, plastic bags, handkerchiefs and children's clothes have been tied. Just beyond this tree lies the 'well', a perfectly formed, round hollow in a large rock, containing a small amount of water and many coins. According to traditional lore there is always water in this *ballán* stone and warts washed in it will disappear.

The Wart Stone lies in rough grass, beside a busy junction known as Rathbride Cross Roads, a few kilometres north of Kildare town. It is an ancient boundary marker for Brigid's (saint and goddess) land on the Curragh; this is a marvellous 2,000 hectare plain of species-rich grassland, which is open, dry and flat, perfect for racing horses on. The Wart Stone is a large, low, roughly square, flat-topped boulder and as the name suggests a cure for warts exists there. Rain pools in a small, natural indentation on the top surface of the rock and unwanted warts should be rubbed with this water. A man who lived nearby told me of the belief; however, I saw little sign of human activity around this historic stone. I think it is rarely used for cures now, but it continues to wait and to watch, as it has done for millennia.

A fascinating group of *ballán* stones is located on the edge of Upper Lough MacNean, near the border village of Blacklion in north Cavan. There is a small, ruined church along the bustling Sligo to Enniskillen road. St Brigid's Stone is sited to the rear of this church, in the corner of a field and next to an unruly hawthorn hedge. It is very close to the lakeshore and the boundary with Northern Ireland which runs through the lough.

I had to search for this stone and eventually came across it partially hidden by blackthorn, briars and bluebells. It is a large rock, almost circular, about 30 cm tall and with a flat surface on top; here, a big, round stone is centrally placed. Around this centre stone nine smaller, smooth, egg-shaped stones sit perfectly in carved-out hollows; the centre stone is not in an indentation, it is flat-bottomed. To the lakeside of this boulder, and touching it, there are two smaller, lower rocks, with a further five *ballán* lying in depressions on them, one large solo stone and a group of four.

This cluster of stones is called after St Brigid, probably because she is believed to have co-founded a Christian community here, but they are more likely to have originated in pagan times. They appear to be almost forgotten, although under one of the stones there were a few coins, indicating that someone had engaged with them relatively recently. I was informed by an elderly, local man that they are 'cursing stones' and he did not recall them ever being used for curing. He said that a curse could be laid by turning the stones anti-clockwise; however, there was a danger that it would backfire on the person making it, if it was not justified!

Inishmurray is a small, low-lying island in the Atlantic, 7 km off the coast of north Sligo. The inhabitants were removed from it in 1948 for practical reasons and re-settled on the mainland. A well-preserved, early Christian monastic settlement remains there, and it is now enjoyed primarily by the birds and the bees, and a few intrepid tourists in the summer months. Inishmurray is famous for its 'cursing stones' or Clocha Breacha as the islanders called them. There are about fifty of these smooth, round stones (some inscribed with crosses and circles); they vary in size and cover an outdoor altar.

Dr Patrick Heraughty was born on Inishmurray and wrote extensively about life on the island, its history and customs. He explained that, 'When an islander wished to bring down vengeance on an enemy, he or she could perform the Big Station in reverse, walking against the sun instead of *deiseal* or clockwise and turning over each of the round stones on *Clocha Breacha* while completing the circuit (typically three rounds of the altar) of that station.' He also warned that a curse laid unjustly would come back to haunt the person who made it. I do not know if people use these stones for this dark purpose anymore, but I think not. Today, visitors to this lovely, untouched island enjoy its simple pleasures, lying on sunny rocks, swimming in cool inlets, and observing the abundance of nature on land, in sky and sea.

# CHAPTER 16

# Holy Wells

A N ESTIMATED 3,000 HOLY WELLS have survived in Ireland according to the *Atlas of the Irish Rural Landscape*. There were probably many more in centuries past. The veneration of these sacred wells has been taking place continuously for at least 2,000 years and possibly for much longer; maybe since the first people came to live on this island 10,000 years ago, and long before the arrival of Christianity. The wells have served both a functional and ritualistic purpose; they were an important source of fresh drinking water for local people and those travelling past, and a place for spiritual expression. Professor Proinsias Mac Cana wrote in 1970 that, 'The cult of wells is, of course, ancient and well attested among the insular Celts and is reflected in the great number of "holy wells" frequented until recent times in Ireland.'

Nowadays the wells vary from simple springs in the earth to elaborately enclosed and decorated structures. Healing and good health have always been strongly linked to these water sources and many holy wells are still associated with specific cures. Water remains a powerful religious symbol in Ireland. The Christian Churches use it for baptisms

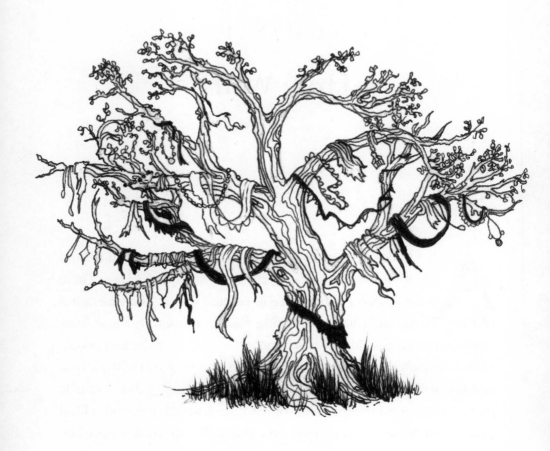

*There are rag trees at many holy wells and people attach personal items*
*to them. The 'rag' is left at the tree, and the person's ill health or problem*
*with it: their illness is transferred to the tree.*

and often there is a holy water font at the entrance to chapels; a splash of this water is part of a blessing.

Over the centuries the early Christians, and later the Catholic Church, incorporated holy wells and other pagan places and celebrations into their religious practice. The sacred sites were gradually and sometimes dramatically assimilated into Christian worship. In particular the royal 'palaces' were built upon or close to them. The Rock of Cashel, the famous twelfth-century ecclesiastical settlement, had been the traditional seat of the Munster kings. Dún Ailinne, not far from the Curragh and Kildare town (St Brigid's territory), was where Leinster was ruled from. A church was placed on the Hill of Tara, the premier pagan location in Ireland, home of the High King and the mysterious Lia Fáil (Stone of Ireland), a large pillar stone.

This Christian assimilation took place most impressively and effectively at Armagh, a short distance from Emain Macha (Navan Fort), the pagan heart of Ulster power. Armagh town or Ard Mhacha, the height of Macha (the war goddess), is where today two cathedrals stand, Catholic and Protestant (Church of Ireland), and it is the location of the archbishops of both Churches. Mac Cana believed 'the druids were the unremitting antagonists of the Church in a long-drawn-out ideological struggle which ended in the virtual annihilation of the druidic organisation'. Logan, in his book on *The Holy Wells of Ireland*, speculated that, 'During the second half of the fifth century, when Christianity was displacing paganism in Ireland the conflict between the old and the new may have been fought out near the sacred wells ... The sign of the victory of the saint was that he blessed the well and used the water to baptise the new Christians.'

Holy wells were important during the penal times (1700s) when Irish Catholics were persecuted. Mass rocks (large, rough, rock altars), situated at some rural holy wells, were where priests tended to their followers in secret and safety. In the 1800s Catholicism became deeply entwined with the ideology of nationalism and with the people's struggle for freedom from the oppression of English colonisation. At this time the Catholic Church tried to control the patron gatherings which took place at holy wells. They saw these festivities as wild and irreverent, and at odds with Christianity. Peter Harbison has written about pilgrimage in Ireland and he recalled the work of the Ordnance Survey men in the 1830s who mapped the country for the British Empire, but who also recorded 'antiquities and folk traditions before the Catholic Church acted to quell the pattern days at holy wells because of the "drunkenness and debauchery" and faction fights which took place in the evenings after the pious practices of the day had been completed'.

Many holy wells are dedicated to particular saints, often little-known, local ones, and a pilgrimage (or patron, *pátrún*, pattern) to the well usually takes place on a specific day. Folklore scholar Máire MacNeill, writing in the 1960s, described the patron as 'an outdoor rural festive gathering with a religious core ... a combination of pilgrimage with festivity ... held once a year on the feast of the patron-saint of the parish ... [which] consisted almost always of rounds with a prescribed set of prayers at the well'. In 1985 Janet and Colin Bord published *Sacred Waters*, an exploration of the holy wells of Britain and Ireland. They wrote that the rituals performed at holy wells ranged from simple to complex, and that, 'The most complex are recorded from those areas where the well cult has survived the longest – Scotland and, especially, Ireland.' The modern concept of a 'wishing' well, which is strong in England, has its origin in the holy well tradition.

When people visit holy wells in Ireland these days, they (unconsciously) combine the two traditions, Christian and pre-Christian, to meet their psychological and spiritual needs. They pray at the well for good health, for success in life and for strength to cope with challenges. They drink the well water and bless themselves with it; they may rub it on a part of their body that needs healing and many take a bottle of this holy water home. A station can be completed too. This is a prescribed ritual of movement and prayer which varies from well to well. The person always moves to the left, clockwise, following the direction of the sun from east to west (*deiseal* in Irish), and generally three, seven or nine circuits of the well are necessary.

The Bords considered the rationale behind this practice of *deiseal* circumambulations of sacred wells. They felt that it was because 'the movement echoed that of the sun … It reflected the need once universally felt to live in harmony with cosmic forces represented in this case by the sun as ultimate generator of life. To circumambulate clockwise was … regarded as life-enhancing and bringing luck.' The station also refers to the different components or physical locations that are part of the ritual, such as the well, and now and then a small cairn of stones known as a 'bed', most likely an ancient ruin or megalithic tomb.

In addition, people regularly partake in the very old custom of attaching a personal item to a rag tree which is a feature of many holy wells. They leave a little bit of themselves or their loved ones at the tree (or well), normally something they are wearing, or have in their handbag or pocket. The rag or offering represents the person who has left it there or the individual they are hoping to help. In the past it was a piece of the person's clothing that was tied to the tree and it was seen as a way in which their illness or troubles could be transferred to the tree, or left at the well.

Anna Rackard recalled in the book *Fish, Stone, Water* (photographs of Irish holy wells), that 'Traditionally, rags were used to wash the afflicted part of the body with water from the well and were then tied to the tree or bush. As the rag deteriorated, the pain faded away … the tree itself "takes on" the pilgrim's pain.' Writing in the latter part of the nineteenth century Lady Wilde stated that, 'There is no superstition stronger in Ireland than a belief in the curative power of the sacred wells ... fountains of health and healing.' She noted that if there was a whitethorn or ash tree at the well, 'the patient ties a votive offering to the branches – generally a coloured handkerchief or a bright red strip cut from a garment; and these offerings are never removed. They remain for years fluttering in the wind and the rain.'

From 2005–10 and continuing in 2017–19, I visited and documented a number of holy wells. These are wells which are frequented by the public, used to help and heal people, and some of them are known for particular cures, such as Tobernalt (possibly *Tobar na nAlt*, well of the body joint), a picturesque holy well on the shore of Lough Gill close to Sligo town. It is situated in a quiet, wooded glade, and a little stream flows continuously from its enclosed spring. St Patrick is reputed to have travelled to this well and to have left the imprint of his fingers in the Mass rock there. People now put their fingers in these holes and pray to the saint for assistance with whatever ails them. Anyone with back pain can also look for a cure on this simple altar, by pressing their back into a natural curve in the rock.

People visit the well every day, to pray, to light candles and to drink the spring water. The mark of man and the Catholic Church is on this holy well, yet it retains its charm and sense of tranquillity. The rag tree above the well is wild and impressive, and harks back to pagan beliefs. It is a small holly bush colourfully laden with a myriad of personal belongings: ribbons, hair bobbles, jewellery, shoelaces, socks, scarves, clothing labels, glasses, keys, strips of plastic, rosary beads, holy medals, monopoly money, children's teddies and women's stockings.

Tadhg Kilgannon, a Sligoman, photographer and antiquarian, had visited The Holy Well (as it is known locally) in the 1920s. On that occasion he was with a friend, a Mr Scallan, who was an officer with the British Expeditionary Forces. When this man came upon the rag tree at Tobernalt, he informed Kilgannon that 'he saw the very same practices being performed by natives at a well a few miles from Khartoum [Sudan]

– tying strips torn from their under garments to bushes there, in order to effect a cure for some malady'.

Another Sligoman, Michael Quirke, understands that today the goddess is to be found in the landscape surrounding this well, in the mountains and ancient cairns, and especially in the waters. Here her three aspects are present; the lake (Lough Gill) is Fiondeabhair the bright girl, the holy well (Tobernalt) is Maeve the powerful woman, and the nearby river (Garavogue) is Garbhóg the wise old woman or *cailleach* who offers immortality.

Tobar Mhuire (Well of Mary) in north Leitrim is a short walk from the village of Killargue. It is in a grove of trees, surrounded by ferns, flowers and birdsong, a peaceful place to contemplate and to be alone. A little wall has been constructed around the holy well which is towered over by a sycamore. Steps lead down to the small, dark spring, lodged between large rocks; lots of coins have been tossed into it. There is a stone shrine adjacent to the well, adorned with holy statues, candles and offerings: plants, sweets, wool, scapulars, necklaces, memorial cards, a baby's soother and a walking stick. From a holly tree close by hang girls' hairbands, bobbles and ribbons, and men's handkerchiefs. A local woman told me that there is no specific cure connected to this well, but that many people seeking healing come here; they pray and drink the water. Mass is held at the holy well every year on 15 August.

Turlough O'Carolan, the celebrated eighteenth-century blind composer and harpist, is buried at Kilronan near Keadue village in north Roscommon. Opposite the cemetery on the shoreline of Lough Meelagh St Lasair's holy well is located. This well is shallow but quite big, with a low wall surrounding it and steps descending to the water. There were a few personal items left at it; little stones and seashells, keyrings, coins, safety pins, a watch and children's sunglasses. I talked to a woman in the graveyard who said that this holy well is regularly visited by the public and that there are two cures linked to it, for warts and a bad back. Next to the spring there is a small, hollowed-out stone embedded in the earth; unwanted warts should be washed in the water which collects in this stone.

St Ronan is remembered as the father of St Lasair and beside the well is the substantial 'Ronan's altar'. It is a large, rectangular slab of rock, supported by four chunky, cut stone pillars and with a big, smooth, oval stone resting on top. There is plenty of room to crawl under the altar and those with back problems must do this to receive the cure. They should crawl from the front to the back of the stone slab and from one side to the other; the movement thereby being made in the shape of a crucifix. Some thoughtful person has made this ritual easier by placing sand and two mats under the altar. Maura Keaveney wrote of this holy well in the 1930s as part of The Schools' Collection; she noted that people went under the flagstone three times to get relief from back pain. They also circled the well three times while praying and took three mouthfuls of well water on each circuit (NFCS 230: 35).

The ruins of the twelfth-century Abbey Assaroe are in a wooded glen to the west of Ballyshannon town in south Donegal. There is an old mill too, a small cave (Catsby) and a little river rushing down to the sea. A tiny holy well can be found on the shore below the abbey. Tobar na Bachaille (well of the crozier) bubbles up into a rock pool and it has ties to St Patrick: he allegedly stamped his foot on this rock and fresh water sprang forth. Five rough, upright rocks (the stations), each topped with an iron cross, have been placed a brief distance apart to form a circle with the well.

A hand-painted sign directs pilgrims to first wash their feet in the sea and to gather fifteen pebbles. Three drinks of water are to be taken from the well, accompanied by a blessing. The person should then walk clockwise around the stations, leaving a pebble and praying (Our Father, Hail Mary and Glory Be) at each one. This ritual must be repeated twice more, and to complete the station a Rosary is said at St Patrick's statue in the adjacent shrine. This popular holy well has a spectacular rag tree; on the day I documented it the lower branches of this ash tree were decorated with socks of every colour, handkerchiefs, dishcloths, tights, shoelaces, ribbons, bracelets, a child's sandal and a green bra!

Father Moore's Well is in the townland of Rathbride (fort of Brigid), 5 km north of Kildare town and close to the previously mentioned Wart Stone. Father Moore was born in 1779 and lived nearby. His holy well, in a quiet rural setting, is visited daily and cared for by the local community. There is a sturdy wall around the well and a homemade message on a wooden blank resting against it reads, 'Do not be anxious all will be well.' Inside the entrance gate a large statue of Mary stands on an altar and under this people have left plants, candles and holy pictures, as well as written requests for assistance from Father Moore.

The holy well is broad, shallow and still, and three big, flat-topped stepping stones have been laid through the centre of it. A modern sign tells visitors of the traditional prayers; first say the Rosary, then cross the stepping stones from north to south, pray for Fr Moore, his parents and yourself, wash any ailment you have with well water, and finally say three Hail Marys. Three visits to the well are recommended, preferably on Fridays or Sundays. I met a young couple with a toddler there who informed me that cures are connected to this man. A certain family has a 'chimney pot' hat which belonged to Father Moore; it was given by him to their ancestor to cure a headache. Almost two hundred years after the priest's death (in 1826) people still use this hat to heal, in particular head problems, by placing it on their head and praying. A typed, laminated page with graphics notified visitors of the forthcoming pilgrimage to this holy well and that in attendance would be Father Moore's hat!

There are two holy wells dedicated to St Brigid on the southern outskirts of Kildare town and both are enjoyed by the public. I have already discussed one of them in relation to its five 'prayer stones'. The lesser-known well is sited just outside the high wall of the Japanese Gardens and beside the National Stud; a good location for this world-renowned racehorse breeding centre, next to the well of a fertility goddess! A short path leads from the road to the spring and the paved area in front of it, which is a place for people to gather, sit and relax. The well is contained within a sunken, circular, stone wall, with steps leading down to it, and the water is tranquil and clean. Coins have been thrown into the holy well and above it, inserted into the wall in 1953, a plaque asks, *A briġid Naoṁta, A Muire na nGaeḋeal, Guiḋ Orainn* (Holy Brigid, Mary of the Gaels, pray for us).

Over this water source leggy willows grow, to which lots of colourful ribbons have been tied, and strips of white plastic, necklaces, hair bobbles and rosary beads. A few candles were left on the wall behind the well, a fabric butterfly, and some memorial cards (remembering the dead, their name and photograph). Despite its position next to a bustling visitor attraction, there is a feeling of separateness and wildness about this well; it is as if the spirit of Brigid is still present.

Another St Brigid well not far from Liscannor in County Clare is one of the best-known holy wells in Ireland, primarily because it is along a major tourist road to the nearby Cliffs of Moher. MacNeill recalled the tradition which connects St Brigid to this well; 'It says that she rested there in her chariot on her way from Connacht to Munster.' By the entrance gate there is a large, glass-encased statue of the saint, robed as a nun, holding her staff and a little model church; she is surrounded by flowers and shrubs. The small well is at the end of a long, whitewashed passage, the floor and roof of which are constructed of cut flagstones. It is a dark, shallow pool, open to the sky, overhung with ivy and fuchsia. At times of heavy rainfall, water gushes into the well from an opening above then disappears quickly via an underground stream.

The most striking feature of this well is that both sides of the passageway to it are completely covered in holy pictures and statues, and countless things left behind by those who have visited. These include lots of small portrait photos, memorial cards, baseball caps, ribbons, scarves, hair ties, bracelets, teddy bears and candles. There are a number of tall statues of Mary draped with rosary beads, scapulars and holy medals. Scraps of handwritten notes are everywhere; they seek help from Brigid to heal sickness, and to give strength in times of bereavement and personal difficulty. To read these messages and to look at the photographs of the dead, especially the young, is touching. It is a public place, but it can also be a very private and powerful experience for those spending time there.

Professor Ian Reader has written about the contemporary Buddhist pilgrimage around the Japanese island of Shikoku. He described the temples along this route and how the pilgrims there leave personal items behind them too, 'notably pictures, copies of sutras, prayer requests, and calling cards ... photographs of themselves ... of loved ones (sometimes deceased) ... staffs, shirts, and hats ... leg braces, corsets, and body supports ... left by pilgrims who had experienced miraculous cures.'

Mám Éan (mountain pass of the birds) holy well nestles on an old route through the Maumturk Mountains of west Galway. Perched on the hill above the pass is a life-size, stone sculpture of St Patrick. He stands on a rocky plinth, hands resting on his staff, a sheep at his feet, strong and steadfast against the rains, the winds and the snows. Mám Éan was most likely a significant location for the celebration of the pre-Christian harvest festival of *Lughnasa*; over the centuries it became more closely associated with Patrick. Máire MacNeill wrote that up to the late 1800s a famous patron was held here annually on the last Sunday of July; 'It was the great gathering of the year for the people of the coastlands of Conamara and the mountainy valleys of the Joyce Country.'

I took a trip to this popular holy well on a warm summer day when the hills were full of singing birds, flowering heathers and contented sheep. A stony trail leads up the mountainside and it takes thirty-five minutes of walking a gradual incline to reach the saddle of the windswept pass (250 m) between rocky peaks. Two low, stone walls line the approach to the little well, which is triangular shaped and wedged among rocks. A cup has been left for thirsty pilgrims and a bowl for thirsty dogs. Some offerings had been carefully placed on the stones above the well: coins, pebbles, rings, ribbons and rosary beads. I spoke with a sheep farmer and asked him were specific cures linked to this spring. He replied in the negative, but smiled and suggested that 'If you pray hard enough, it will probably work!'

Leaba Phádraig (Patrick's bed) is to be found on the hillside overlooking the well. It is a recess in the cliff face and a place to shelter from the elements, or in good weather to enjoy splendid views. MacNeill cited folklore gathered in 1942 which recorded that 'those who have lost their health lie on the bed in the hope of being cured'. To the rear of the adjacent modern altar people have left objects which are significant to them: jewellery, teddies, candles, turf and memorial cards. One photograph was of a New York fireman who had died in the 9/11 tragedy (2001).

In contrast to the dramatic, mountain setting of Mám Éan holy well, St Augustine's Well is almost in the centre of Galway. It is on the shore of a minor estuary known as Lough Atalia (Loch an tSáile, lake of salt water), to the east of the city and along a very busy road. The name derives from its connection to the Augustinian priory nearby. This holy well is tidal and sea water covers it twice daily; the depth of water varies from day to day with the tides. A flight of rocky steps descends from the road to the shoreline, where relatively recently a stone altar and cross were installed, along with information on the history of the well. I saw few personal belongings left there, probably because they are washed away by the sea.

The well is small and shallow, with plenty of pebbles and some coins in it, and is surrounded by a low, hexagonal, whitewashed wall.

Another stone wall encircles this, with a third row of rocks defining the perimeter; all the walls are low, offering least resistance to the tide. An opening in the wall and two rows of stone direct the water flowing from the spring down to the lough, where a white, concrete cross has been erected. An unusual, circular stone is at the base of this cross, carved with a crucifix and the letters IHS (a Christogram meaning Jesus). The holy well is overlooked by apartments and houses. There is continuous traffic noise, and people rushing past, absorbed in their lives, and the water from this little well keeps quietly flowing, as it has for thousands of years.

I knocked on a handful of doors in the vicinity and was told by a helpful, middle-aged woman that this holy well remains popular with the public. It has a cure for eye ailments; splash the well water onto the eyes and face. She said people take the spring water home with them and that there used to be a lot more coins in the well, but people take them home too! The Bords noted that a cure for sore eyes was attached to many holy wells and this they speculated was because 'in earlier centuries eye troubles were more frequent ... perhaps caused by smoky cottage interiors?'

Beside the village of Fore in County Westmeath there are the substantial ruins of a medieval Benedictine abbey. The first monastery was founded at Fore (*fobhar*, a well or spring) in the seventh century by a Sligo nobleman, St Féichín. Today people visit his holy well there in search of cures, particularly for headache and toothache. The day I called by this well was virtually dry. From the centre of it grew a small ash tree which was heavily laden with rags: socks, strips of fabric, hair bobbles, shoelaces, plastic bags, sweet wrappers and empty crisp packets. Coins had been hammered into the tree's bark and numerous ones cast into the well. It is said that timber from this tree will not burn, nor will water from the well boil. There is a second rag tree a short distance away on the site of a former vat, where according to the information sign, 'Delicate children were immersed in the water to obtain a cure through the invocation of St Feichin.'

A glance at a map shows that this early Christian settlement is but 9 km cross-country from the mighty megalithic cemetery of Loughcrew, near Oldcastle, County Meath. In Irish Loughcrew is known as Sliabh na Caillí, the hill of the witch (the goddess), and over twenty-five passage tombs (cairns) are concentrated on four hills there; they are believed to be 5,000 years old. The establishment of Fore as an important site of Christian worship so close to this pagan centre of power is unlikely to have been accidental.

Tobar na nGealt (well of the crazy) is located not far from the village of Camp in west Kerry. Having heard of the well's reputation for curing mental health problems, I went to find it. Just off a quiet country road and tucked behind unchecked bushes and ferns, this holy well could easily be missed. However, a hand-painted board, fixed to a roadside tree, bears its name. A muddy path leads to the well, which when I visited looked more like a stream, emerging from under the road and channelling water from the mountain valley above to the sea below.

The goat willow overhanging the well has become its rag tree, with bracelets, necklaces, ribbons, feathers, shells and a child's toy advertising a fast-food chain all tied randomly to its straggling branches. I talked to a friendly farmer in the locality and she informed me that there is a spring under the stream. She understands that this has been a sacred and healing well for millennia, and that the seventh-century king known as Mad Sweeney had found peace following the drinking of its water.

Patrick Logan alluded to writings on this well from the 1830s, where it was stated that those looking for a cure drank the water and ate the cress growing there, and 'They give many instances of mad persons who sojourned in this valley, and returned home, sane and in excellent health.' As a result of their research into holy wells, Janet and Colin

Bord asserted that, 'There can be little doubt that people do sometimes find cures at healing wells.' They put forward two possible reasons for why these cures occur: '1. the water does contain something which acts upon the body; or 2. the patient's own intrinsic healing abilities are stimulated by visiting the well.' They also felt that people who went to holy wells hoping for cures 'clearly believed that the wells had the power to cure, and the long survival of holy wells demonstrates the strength of this belief'.

The Chink Well is in a sea cave and is covered at high tide. It is at Portrane, 20 km north of Dublin city and close to the town of Donabate. From Tower Bay beach car park, a short cliff walk to the south commences. Follow it for five minutes until you come to the third rocky cove along this trail; it is directly below the unmissable nineteenth-century round tower. Before reaching the high wall and fence which enclose the narrow path descend over the rocks to the beach. But be warned, this holy well should only be accessed at low tide as there is a danger of getting trapped by the incoming sea.

There are a few caves in the cove. The first one is tall, narrow and deep; to the rear of the cave there is a tunnel, the opening of which is about 5 m above the sand and therefore difficult to enter. It is known as the Priest's Chamber and it was documented by Thomas Byrne in the 1930s as a place where persecuted Catholic clergy hid during the penal times; his account is part of The Schools' Collection (NFCS 789: 271). Adjacent there is a second cave, which is more of a big, open cleft in the cliff face, tapering inwards. At the back of this cave water flows steadily from a gap under the cliff, across a boulder and lodges briefly in two rock pools. The water in the pool closest to the mouth of the cave forms a small, natural 'well'.

This is a tranquil place to sit for a while, looking across the bay to Ireland's Eye and Howth Head, and listening to the sounds of the seashore. I believe this holy well is rarely visited nowadays, but if someone were to go there in need of healing, I think they would bless themselves, say some prayers, and wash the affected area with water from the well. Dr Logan wrote in 1980 that it was thought this holy well had the cure of whooping cough (also known as chin cough, which may be the reason for the well's name, chink), and that, 'People seeking a cure leave all sorts of votive offerings at it, so that they may be swept out to sea on the next ebb tide, and if this is seen to occur a favourable result is expected.'

Colman mac Duagh's Well is in the heart of the Burren National Park in north Clare. It is a beautiful holy well, hidden in hazel scrub and towered over by the cliffs of Slieve Carran. You must take an ancient trackway across fields of limestone 'pavement' to reach the little, ruined church. This is where Colman, a sixth-century ascetic saint, lived and prayed for seven years in solitude. On the hillside above there is a cave where folklore says he slept. The entrance, a dark triangular opening, is reminiscent of a chapel door. The space inside is small and womb-like, with just enough room for a tall man to lie down.

The holy well is on the slope below the church. A circular, stone wall frames it and in this a gap has been left to allow ease of access. Some water from the stream which rushes past the well is diverted into it, thereby creating a shallow pool within the walls. A few shells and coins rest in this water, and a handful of ribbons are tied to the neighbouring bushes. Just uphill of the well the stream emerges from under the mountain; its water is cold and crystal clear. All around there is an abundance of ferns, mosses cloak the rocks and lichens thrive on the trees. I visited this holy well on a sunny spring day, and left with a strong sense of the enduring presence of the natural world, of the simplicity of life, and of peace.

Elizabeth Healy, in her book *In Search of Ireland's Holy Wells*, has written that:

The cult of the wells could not have endured so long unless it satisfied some deep-felt need in our consciousness ... The offerings left at wells seem to reflect every need of human existence: for health, for fertility, for jobs, for houses, for a good partner in life, for family harmony ... the prayers repeated like a mantra ... serve to focus the mind ... allows our own healing powers to come into play ... to bring peace to mind and soul ... [we] carry out the prescribed rituals, and have the satisfaction of knowing we have participated in a ceremony that connects us to our deepest and oldest roots.

## Save a Well

There are thousands of wells across Ireland, some known as holy wells, others simply as sources of spring water. Many wells are now neglected and forgotten. If you know of a local well that needs care and attention, I would encourage you to be proactive, to clear around it, to clean it out and to tend to it. Remember those who have gone before us, who depended on this source, who respected and protected it; and let us never forget that water is life.

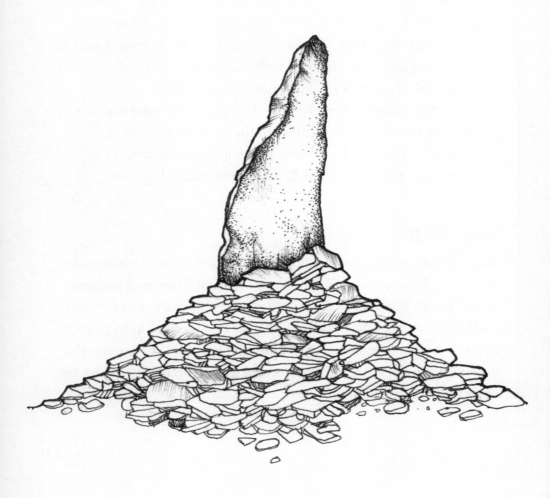

*Mount Brandon, in west Kerry, is associated with the sixth-century*
*St Brendan. Cosán na Naomh, one path to the summit, is marked*
*regularly by small cairns of stone. This is a wonderful walk.*

# CHAPTER 17

# Pilgrimage

The celebration of Garland Sunday takes place on the last Sunday in July and today religious ceremonies are held at some holy wells. This special day at the end of the summer is the Christian assimilation of the pagan beginning-of-harvest festival, *Lughnasa* (*Lúnasa* is August in Irish); it honoured the sun god Lugh who had the power to ensure a successful harvest. Lugh, a god of the Celts, was worshipped across Europe and the city of Lyon in eastern France is understood to be named after him. He is known as the hero of the second Battle of Moytura (in south-east Sligo) because he killed his tyrannical grandfather Balor of the Evil Eye. He did this with a sling shot through the giant's eye and thereby ensured victory for the Tuatha Dé Danann over the Fomorians. It is said that when Balor's venomous eye hit the earth a large hole was created, which subsequently filled with water, and it became the nearby Lough Nasool (*loch na súile*, lake of the eye).

The fairies have dominated Irish folklore; the leprechaun played a minor role. This small, mischievous man has received greater attention in recent decades and is now synonymous with the international marketing of our country! Leprechaun or *luchorpán* could be translated as 'Lugh of the little body'. Wood carver Michael Quirke believes that the leprechaun character may be a representation of Lugh, and that this was a way in which the old pagan god was diminished and ridiculed, and thereby weakened in his power and resistance to the new Christian God.

The festival of *Lughnasa* (Lugh assembly/games) or Garland Sunday had different names around the country, Crom Dubh's Sunday, Fraochán/Bilberry Sunday or Lammas Sunday. Crom Dubh featured strongly in the tales from the west; Ó hÓgáin described him as the 'archetypal pagan in folk tradition, represented as an opponent of Patrick in that saint's mission ... usually called Crom Dubh ... "dark croucher", an image of the devil'.

In the nineteenth and early twentieth centuries community celebration of the harvest was still a highlight of the year for country people, who put on their Sunday best and headed to the hills, springs, lake and seashores, to eat, drink, sing and court. Folklorist Bríd Mahon recalled that a 1942 questionnaire about Garland Sunday got a huge response. People outlined how they 'celebrated the beginning of the harvest by making trips to hills, mountains and lakes ... They picked bilberries and wild fruit, ate the first of the new potatoes ... drank homemade wine and poteen, told stories and danced the night away to the music of the fiddle.'

Eloquently written and meticulously researched, *The Festival of Lughnasa* was published by Máire MacNeill in 1962 and she too used the folklore collected twenty years earlier as the basis for her book. She wrote that:

> Lughnasa is in its essence the festival of the first fruits of the tilled fields ... the day when the sickle was first put to the ripened corn ... the spade turned up the first meal of potatoes

... the securing of the main food supply ... [or as an old woman from Ballinrobe had put it] 'The harvest is in and the hunger is over!'

Brian Friel's play *Dancing at Lughnasa* is set in the glens of south Donegal (August 1936) in the poor but happy home of the five unmarried Mundy sisters. The harvest is the backdrop to this story of a family on the cusp of great change and references to the celebration of the festival of *Lughnasa* are skilfully interwoven. Innocent Rose recounts to her sisters, 'It was last Sunday week, the first night of the Festival of Lughnasa; and they were doing what they do every year up there in the back hills ... First they light a bonfire beside a spring well. Then they dance around it. Then they drive their cattle through the flames to banish the devil out of them.'

## Croagh Patrick

Garland Sunday is the day of the famous annual pilgrimage to Croagh Patrick (the Reek) in County Mayo. This striking, conical-shaped mountain, at the edge of the Atlantic Ocean, rises to 765 m. On this day up to 25,000 people from the west of Ireland and beyond, and from every walk of life, follow the centuries-old tradition of climbing the holy mountain. 'Dawn breaks secretly as the great human snake weaves up the mountainside.'

Their *turas* or journey winds slowly and often painfully up and up to the barren, rocky summit and the small, white church. Throughout the day women, men and children join in a collective struggle to the top, sticks in hand, resolute, defiant of the wind, the rain, the sun and the steep, dangerous path. As they walk (some barefoot) they pray for themselves and for those they love; they pray for good physical and mental health, for healing from serious illness, for help with personal problems, for deceased family and friends, and they give thanks for what has brought them happiness. For each person the experience is individual, yet there is also a strong sense of community and shared support, a friendly greeting, a kind word of encouragement, a welcome drink of water.

When I climbed Croagh Patrick on Reek Sunday I was struck by the sight of a very elderly woman, attired in headscarf, skirt and sandals, being gently walked back down the rock-strewn path by three young, brightly clad mountain rescue volunteers. The portraits in *Atlantic Tabor: The Pilgrims of Croagh Patrick* (2016), were taken on Reek Sunday over a five-year period by two Polish photojournalists, Tomasz Bereska and Tomasz Szustek, and they capture the atmosphere, the diversity of people and the humanity at the core of this special pilgrimage.

Croagh Patrick has possibly been a sacred mountain for thousands of years and it was probably an important pre-Christian site for the celebration of *Lughnasa*. It was the mountain where St Patrick (fifth century) supposedly lived, fasted and prayed for forty days. He is believed to have battled with the devil's mother here, who was sometimes described as a great serpent, dragon or worm (*ollphéist*). This legend and that of Patrick banishing the snakes from Ireland can be seen as covert portrayals of the victory of the new patriarchal religion and God over the old worship of multiple deities, and in particular over the goddess. The serpent is the Goddess or Earth Mother, the source of all life, and of the endless natural cycle of birth, death and rebirth. MacNeill discussed Christianity's suppression of paganism with reference to Croagh Patrick; I have expanded on her train of thought in my exploration of the number seven.

Lady Wilde noted, 'We are told also by the ancient chroniclers that serpent-worship once prevailed in Ireland, and that St Patrick hewed down the serpent idol ... the great worm ... from whence arose the legend that St Patrick banished all venomous things from the island.'

Patrick Logan was aware that 'a contest between saint and serpent' was a story linked to many of the Irish saints. It was written that when St Kevin came to Glendalough, he 'was able to displace a serpent which lived in the Upper Lake and did harm to men and beasts, but the saint moved it to the Lower Lake, where it did no further harm'.

Mary Condren's thought-provoking book *The Serpent and the Goddess* explores in depth this gradual but seismic shift in Ireland from polytheism to monotheism. She writes that, 'Crushing the serpent/ Goddess, therefore, symbolized the overthrow of those societies, together with their religions, which were matricentered.' The *Dictionary of the Celts* states that, 'In Celtic Mythology and belief, the snake was associated with fertility and with healing and also with the Otherworld.' I note that a symbol used by pharmacies in Ireland today is a snake entwining a goblet, known as the Bowl of Hygieia; she was a Greek goddess of health.

An ancient road led directly west from Rathcroghan (the royal seat of pagan Connacht and home of Queen Maeve), on the verdant plains of Roscommon, to the holy mountain. The latter part of this route, 35 km from the thirteenth-century Ballintubber Abbey to Croagh Patrick, has become a walking trail for pilgrims. It is known as *Tóchar Phádraig* (Patrick's causeway) and meanders through the Mayo countryside. It was from Rathcroghan (now a landscape rich in archaeological monuments), close to the village of Tulsk, that the epic *Táin Bó Cúailnge* began. Legend tells us that Maeve wanted a bull to equal her husband Ailill's, so she went to war with Ulster and stole their magnificent Brown Bull of Cooley.

These days Maeve (Medb or Medhbh) is remembered as a troublesome queen, reputedly buried upright facing her enemies in an impressive cairn atop Knocknarea on the Sligo coastline; Knocknarea was traditionally translated as *cnoc na rí*, hill of the king, but it could be *cnoc na ré*, hill of the moon. In pre-Christian times Maeve was worshipped as the goddess of sovereignty, bringing stability, fertility and prosperity to the land. Proinsias Mac Cana wrote in *Celtic Mythology* of 'manifestations of the earth-goddess, who are primarily associated with the land in all its various aspects: its fertility, its sovereignty, its embodiment of the powers of death as well as of life ... The concept of the land of Ireland as a goddess was deeply rooted and it did not die easily.'

There is a cave, Uaimh na gCat (cave of the cats), at Rathcroghan which was considered to be a way into the Otherworld. The Morrígan (*mór ríoghain*, great queen), the war goddess, resided here and young warriors had to spend time in this underground chamber as part of their initiation rites. I visited this cave with a local guide. Down a rutted lane, in a little field, there is a small, unremarkable opening underneath a large slab of rock and a hawthorn bush. You slither through, passing an ogham stone inscribed (using a series of lines) *of Fráech son of Medb*, into a short, stone-lined passageway. The cave is long and narrow, tall and airy, a natural fissure in the soft limestone. It is cool, black dark and silent.

## Lough Derg

St Patrick's Purgatory, or Lough Derg (as it is commonly known), has been a place of Christian pilgrimage for over 1,000 years. It is a complex of buildings covering the small, flat Station Island in a remote corner of south-east Donegal. Lough Derg can be translated as *loch dearg*, the red lake, which may refer to the blood of the mighty worm or water serpent that St Patrick is said to have killed here, having followed her from Croagh Patrick. American anthropologist Walter Evans Wentz visited the area in 1909 and collected tales; he discovered that 'the old men and women in this neighbourhood used to believe that Lough Derg was the last stronghold of the Druids in Ireland; and from what I have heard them say, I think the old legend means that this is where St Patrick ended his fight with the Druids, and that the serpents represent the Druids or paganism'.

Derg might also be *deirc*, a hole or hollow, alluding to a cave on the island which was thought to be an entrance to hell. In medieval times pilgrims travelled from all over Europe to the island and this cave (this 'purgatory', a place of cleansing), to pray and fast for fifteen days. In her book *The Archaeology of Caves in Ireland* Dr Marion Dowd recalls:

> a pilgrimage made there by an English knight named Owein in 1146 or 1147. During his 24-hour solitary stay in the cave, the knight witnessed devils torturing sinners ... He also received visions of a paradise brimming with flowers and perfumes ... This account of the knight's experiences achieved enormous popularity across Medieval Europe ... It appears to have influenced Dante's *Divine Comedy*.

Laurence Flynn described how the pilgrimage was twice suppressed, in 1632 (part of England's colonisation of Ireland) with 'the destruction of everything on the island ... including the original cave', and in 1704 when an Act of Parliament 'imposed a fine of ten shillings or a public whipping as penalty for resorting to such places of pilgrimage'. Today no remnant of the cave survives; it is thought to be under the foundations of the modern basilica or maybe the bell tower mound.

About 11,000 people (primarily Catholics) visit Lough Derg every summer and many of them make the three-day pilgrimage, as I did. This involves going barefoot, an overnight vigil, two dawn Masses and fasting; the only sustenance is water, black tea and dry bread. At the centre of this pilgrimage is the station (a lengthy ritual of repetitive prayer and movement) and nine of these must be completed over the three days. It takes place mostly outdoors at the 'penitential beds' (the remains of early Christian, stone beehive cells) and around the basilica. The flow of people is slow and continuous. They shuffle along, whispering their prayers, absorbed in their thoughts, and struggling with fatigue, hunger, cold, rain and midges.

Lough Derg is a unique place in twenty-first-century Ireland. It is a place of quiet (mobile phones are forbidden), a place to pray, to reflect and to be at peace. Lots of the people who make the pilgrimage do so for an 'intention'; they are looking for help with their problems, or those of their family and friends. Often, they come to pray for the healing of someone they love. One woman I spoke to told me that she was there for her brother-in-law who was very sick with cancer; another was wishing her sister-in-law could conceive and bear a healthy child; some prayed for their children's success in state exams.

When people are at Lough Derg, they are kind, friendly and open, and they talk; strangers will tell you their life story. This pilgrimage is a deeply personal experience, a challenge for each individual, physically and mentally. But there is a feeling as well of collective sharing of the difficulties encountered, and mutual comfort and strength comes from moving and praying as a group. As we boarded the boat on the third morning some people were quiet, tired and relieved, others were chatty, laughing and feeling fabulous!

## Mount Brandon

Another holy mountain is Brandon on the spectacular Dingle Peninsula in west Kerry; this pilgrimage is lesser-known than the one to Croagh Patrick. Mount Brandon's summit (953 m) is highly likely to have been a site of pagan worship, including for the *Lughnasa* celebration. Now it is associated with the sixth-century saint, Brendan; a local holy man who is understood to have spent time on this mountain in solitude and prayer.

I climbed Brandon following the well-trodden Cosán na Naomh (path of the saint), starting in the townland of Baile Breac. There is an elaborate, stone shrine to Mary here, two giant, rock pillars which pilgrims pass between, and a memorial with the names of a few of those who have hiked this route in recent years in search of a cure for cancer 'on the saint's trail protected by Saint Brendan', the inscription reads. This is a wonderful walk. A little path over grass and rock weaves up and up, marked regularly by small cairns of stone topped with tall, numbered, wooden crosses, the fourteen Stations of the Cross. I walked alone. On the lower slopes I enjoyed panoramic views to the south of the Blasket Islands and the expanse of ocean. Then the mist descended and with it an otherworldly atmosphere; all was quiet and peaceful.

The top of this mountain is rock-strewn, windswept and desolate. Máire MacNeill, following her visit there in the 1960s, recounted that:

> On the highest part of the mountain ... a little oratory was built. Its ruins still stand. It is known as Teampaillín Bréanainn (Brendan's little church) ... A few yards away is Tobar Bréanainn (Brendan's Well), beside which there are a number of small mounds known as Na h-Uaigheanna (the Graves). Nearby there also stands a pillar stone called Leac na nDrom (the Stone of the Backs). This mountain sanctuary was formerly a place of pilgrimage.

Today, a large, metal cross and an ordnance survey trig point can be found there too, and the holy well is just a small, water-filled, grassy hollow.

I took the old pilgrim trail on the south-west slope of the mountain, but many others approach it from the eastern side, which is a more strenuous climb, beginning near the village of An Clochán (Cloghane). The traditional patron in honour of St Brendan was held here, and

MacNeill wrote that, 'The Patron of Cloghane was the great assembly of the year in the Dingle Peninsula.' This harvest celebration was revived in 1995 as Féile Lughnasa; it takes place over the last weekend of July, and in 2018 it was promoted on the community website as a festival featuring music, stage dramas, swimming races, blessing of the boats, sheep shearing, a poker tournament and a pilgrimage to the summit of Mount Brandon!

In addition to being a saint, Brendan, known as 'the navigator', was also a great sailor and explorer. In the shadow of the holy mountain nestles Cuas an Bhodaigh (Brandon creek). Legend holds that Brendan and his monks departed from here to sail across the Atlantic and look for the Promised Land. Seven years later they discovered North America, 950 years before Columbus. Over the summers of 1976 and 1977 sailor, historian and adventurer Tim Severin recreated this amazing 7,200 km voyage, in a small, open, leather-hulled boat. Using the Stepping Stone Route via Scotland, the Faroe Isles, Iceland and Greenland, he and his brave crew of four, after sixteen weeks at sea, finally made landfall in Newfoundland, Canada.

## Walk for Health, Healing and Hope

English nature writer Richard Mabey recovered from severe depression by immersing himself in the natural world and falling in love. In his memoir *Nature Cure* he explains, 'The idea of a "nature cure" goes back as far as written history. If you expose yourself to the healing currents of the outdoors, the theory goes, your ill-health will be rinsed away. The Romans had a saying, "solvitur ambulando", which means, roughly, "you can work it out by walking".'

The Camino de Santiago is an extremely popular pilgrimage and walking route across northern Spain. It is estimated that 300,000 people walk parts or all of it annually and they come from every corner of our planet, including lots from Ireland. Each person has their own reasons for embarking on this challenging journey, usually a mixture of religious/spiritual, psychological and physical ones. For more than a millennium, pilgrims have been making their way to Santiago de Compostela by different trails to worship at the shrine of St James, the apostle. His remains are believed to rest in the crypt of the cathedral there. In the past many Irish pilgrims started their journey at St James' Gate in Dublin and sailed to A Coruña, 75 km north of Santiago.

I have walked the Camino Francés route from the little town of Saint-Jean-Pied-de-Port in the French Pyrenees, over snowy mountain passes and raging rivers, through lush vineyards and sleepy pastoral lands, along woodland paths and winding city lanes, past ugly industrial zones and noisy highways, through medieval villages and ancient fortified towns, to eventually reach the Holy Grail of Santiago. I walked the Camino in three sections, coming and going to it, a total of five weeks' walking and 777 km.

When you walk day after day, carrying as light a backpack as you allow yourself, your body enters a new rhythm, it acquires a new level of fitness and a new sense of freedom. I loved when I saw a mountain range in the distance, three days later I was crossing it, and in another three days it was well behind me. This was how people would have travelled in the past, very close to nature, relying on their bodies and wits to make a journey; it felt empowering. On the Camino your mind also enters a new and peaceful space. As the kilometres are eaten up so too are your worries; they start to fade and disappear, and are replaced by simpler, practical concerns like protecting your feet, keeping cool, finding food, a clean bed, a hot shower and washing your socks.

Another outstanding feature of this pilgrimage is the people you meet along the way – Spanish people who are friendly and kind, who help you when lost, serve you graciously, and offer the endless trail of *peregrinos* an encouraging *Buen Camino!* Unforgettable also are the people from all around the world, speaking a myriad of languages, who share their food, their advice and sometimes their stories with you; young women in love and hopeful for the future, parents and their adult children reconnecting, and old men grateful that they had survived the Holocaust. And when you finally arrive in the holy city, weary, relieved and happy, the Catholic Church gives you a certificate of completion, a *compostela*, and (traditionally) the promise of a quicker entry to heaven!

In his writings on the Croagh Patrick pilgrimage, Patrick Claffey, of Trinity College Dublin, refers to Buddhist pilgrims walking clockwise around Mount Kailash (Kangri Rinpoche) in Tibet, one of the most sacred mountains in the world. I have travelled to the holy city of Lhasa, high up in the remote, harsh and vast Himalayas. At the heart of the rambling, vibrant old town is the iconic Jokhang Temple. Devotees from every part of Tibet converge on this place of worship, some of them having walked more than 1,200 km from Mount Kailash. From dawn to dusk they move as one, making slow circumambulations of the temple sunwise, reciting their prayers and rotating their beads. At regular intervals the throng of pilgrims must part to avoid the groups of armed Chinese soldiers who block their way and keep them under continuous surveillance.

I was unable to talk to these people as I did not speak their language, but I think the reasons why they made this pilgrimage were probably similar to those of the Irish and individuals all over the world who embark on spiritual journeys, for their faith, for good health, for healing (often against the odds), for strength to face life's difficulties, to remember their dead, to seek forgiveness for their wrongdoings, and in gratitude for the blessings in their lives.

# CHAPTER 18

# The Future for Cures

🌿

THE TRADITIONAL CURES HAVE SURVIVED in Ireland, particularly in rural areas, as my research has shown. But will they continue to do so? I believe that the cures have strengths which will help them to live on, primarily their ability to change. Cures are adapted to the historical and social context within which they exist, highlighted by the use of new technology and media by those who make and receive cures. However, some cures face serious challenges, such as the falling fertility rate, changes in birth management, the all-pervasive fear of litigation, and the huge threat to plant life.

There was mixed opinion among those I interviewed as to whether the traditional cures are surviving or dying, and what future they have. The majority believed that they are holding on and some felt there was a revival of interest in cures; a minority thought they are dying out, being less used, especially by the younger generation.

## Surviving/Dying

An elderly man in south Leitrim with a cure for colic helped animals

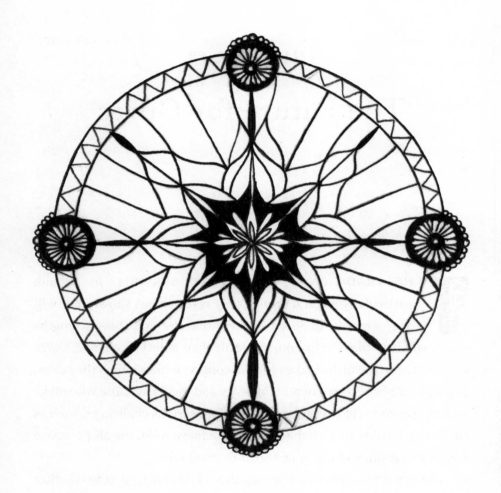

*And we must always remember that each one of us is connected by the great web of Life, and that we share and depend on the natural world, fragile, beautiful and powerful.*

and humans. He and his wife believed the old cures had survived well in their region, 'very much in Leitrim'. A seventh son in County Sligo, who helped those with ringworm, speculated that the cures were being more utilised, 'a full circle, they are coming back, people believe in them'. A woman in south Donegal with an asthma cure knew that there were numerous cures alive and well in her corner of Ireland. She said that 'a lot of people are going for cures, rather than going to the doctor' and that they wanted to avoid taking antibiotics. And a faith healer believed that 'the cures will always survive, once they work'. He felt that many people were looking for alternatives to conventional medicine, that they were interested in a more 'holistic approach to life' and that they were 'beginning to seek out people like myself'.

On the other side of the debate, a man who had the cure of the burn was worried that the cures were dying out. He believed (as I do) that the future of the Irish cure lies with our young people, the next generation, with their willingness to hold on to and utilise the traditional cures. An eighteen-year-old in South Sligo made a cure for bad backs and she thought that the old cures were not being used by most young folk; 'there's a reason they are there ... but people just don't see it,' she said. A retired Leitrim man with a mumps cure was aware of other cures in the county, yet he lamented that in general they were on the decline. 'A lot will only ... go for some cures as a last resort ... for most things now there's medical attention ... They'd be dying out ... with the old generation.'

## Strengths of the Cure
### Adaptation

Cures are traditional, but they are not static. Like every other aspect of life, movement and change takes place in cures, over the years and with each generation. Cures are tweaked and adapted to meet the needs of those making and receiving them; they reflect the society they serve. Small changes occur which do not affect the integrity of the cure but which are meaningful and helpful to those connected to it, and contribute to its survival. Patrick Logan understood that cures were susceptible to change, and he noted that 'folk medicine, like official medicine, tends to discard forms of treatment when something more efficient becomes available'.

Examples of the way in which some cures had been subtly adjusted include one for erysipelas. It was made by an elderly woman and she told me that the man who gave her the cure thirty years previously had instructed her to break up the herb 'with a stone'. She winked and said, 'I have a mixer ... and I stick it into it, and it chops it up grand and fine.' Another younger woman with a sprain cure explained that it involved a short ritual of touch and prayer, repeated three times. She blessed herself between the three parts of the cure, whereas her grandmother had walked away from and returned to the injured person each time. 'Granny used to always walk away ... walk to the door and then walk back again, but we (she and her sisters) don't do that ... We just bless ourselves and start again.'

I interviewed a man who made his cures for headaches and heart problems over three days. He administered the cures after dark, though he knew that 'you're supposed to make them between sunrise and sunset, but I think the sun is shining someplace in the world the whole time'. And a man who had a Bell's palsy cure met those he helped three times over a nine-day period. However, now and then someone was unable to return for the final visit and if they had a good reason, he would make the cure twice for them on the second day. 'If they can't make the third visit, because they're flying back to England ... or America ... then you can do the charm twice, with a small interval in between, on the second visit.'

There was a cattle dealer with a popular cure for bleeding. He had a sprain cure too, a special prayer recited three times, along with three blessings; these prayers were repeated for three days. In the past this cure was only made on Thursdays and Mondays, but he had adapted it; 'I've started to do it any day of the week ... I have so much belief in it.' Also, the person had to come three times to have the sprained area touched by him. However, if they lived a long distance away, they no longer had to be physically present; he would just say the prayers for them. 'I have found ... people far away ... sprained their ankle ... or wrist ... I started to do it for them on the Monday and Thursday, and it has worked ... even if I don't see them.'

## Use of Technology and Local Radio

Mobile phones have become indispensable to contemporary Irish life. They are one of the main ways in which we communicate, conduct our business and social lives. They (and landlines) are also important to traditional healing practice. When needed, friends, family and work colleagues will text or email each other the names, locations and phone numbers of those with cures. People regularly telephone and make enquiries about a cure (or arrange an appointment) before they travel to get it. Those who need a cure urgently, such as to stop bleeding, use their phone to request it, and because the person with the cure will invariably have a mobile, they are accessible at all times. A fisherman with a bleeding cure occasionally received calls in the middle of the night; 'with mobile phones now ... people can get you day and night ... I would answer me phone always.' Reflecting the popularity of mobile phones, credit for them is sometimes given as a gift, in thanks for a cure.

A man who made a prayer cure for a foreign body in the eye said people used to come to his house, but in recent years this happened less. 'I do more phone calls now.' He was farming during the day, so it was best if they called him at home in the evening on the landline.

Another man had a similar eye cure and he normally got asked for it by telephone. He told me that people did not like to leave a message on the answer machine and that they would call back to speak to him in person. His daughter worked in the United Arab Emirates and he had phone calls from there looking for his cure.

An asthma cure I investigated was accompanied by written instructions regarding the procedure to follow and the prayers to say. This was a well-known cure, so in order to reduce the workload, the man making it had typed the information into his computer and every time he made a cure, he printed it out. A full-time healer had a website dedicated to her work; she and one other faith healer that I interviewed utilised the internet in this way. Ten years earlier a person that she had cured of psoriasis set up the website for her; he felt 'more people should know about this all over the world'. She found it a practical help, as it saved her a lot of time repeatedly explaining to people what she did; it is 'easier for them to look, than me explain it on the phone ... then they usually do it [the cure] by post'.

Local radio stations in the west and north-west broadcast the names and telephone numbers of some people with cures. This is often done in response to requests for information on specific cures, and listeners phone in and make suggestions, or recount their experiences of cures live on air. A seventh daughter in Mayo informed me that most heard about her skin cures in the old-fashioned way, by word of mouth; however, the local radio station had her details too and would give them out to the public.

## Challenges for the Cure
*Falling Fertility Rates and Breech Births*

The fertility rate in Ireland has been steadily falling for the past fifty years. Modern records show that the rate peaked in 1965 at just over four births per woman; in 2016 it was less than two (a European norm), and the government expects it to fall to 1.6 by 2031. This demographic trend has major implications for the survival of the seventh daughter/ son healing tradition. It is now rare for an Irish woman to have seven children and the chance of giving birth to seven consecutive girls or boys is becoming extremely unlikely. The cures associated with these individuals will cease to exist, unless something unexpected happens in the future. Some say a seventh son of a seventh son is a powerful healer, but I did not come across anyone who fell into this grouping. Probably, in years gone by, when families were consistently very large, children were born with this status.

I spoke to a twenty-two-year-old who had a ringworm cure because she was a seventh daughter. Many had travelled long distances across Ireland to her home in Sligo to receive the cure. 'They can't seem to find anyone with the cure for the ringworm [where they live]; there's not really big families these days.' She felt that her category of cure could not continue; 'it's definitely going to die out, which is unfortunate'. And a seventh son faith healer in south Leitrim was similarly aware that this healing tradition is in decline: 'It's dead, it's gone, it's history.'

In the past 3–4 per cent of Irish babies were born breech and these people were believed to have a back cure. Nowadays breech delivery is generally considered high risk, therefore foetuses are turned in the womb in late pregnancy or increasingly delivered by caesarean section. Consequently, a breech birth has become an unusual event in Irish hospitals. As the number of breech births diminishes, so too does the chance of survival for this cure.

A Donegal woman with an asthma cure told me that her young daughter also had a cure, for sore backs. Interestingly, this child was born by caesarean section as she was breech; however, she still had the cure. Maybe this belief is a lifeline for the cure of back pain. I think that the parents of girls and boys who were determined to come into this world feet first, but modern medicine intervened to alter their course, can take it that their child has this cure.

## Fear of Litigation

Ireland has become a prosperous country and our new-found wealth has brought with it the need for insurance, in its many forms. Financial awards for personal injury and medical negligence claims are numerous, and often large. The public perception is that a compensation culture exists, with exaggerated and fraudulent claims being common, awards too high, and as a result insurance premiums keep rising. The reality of the situation is difficult to verify as many cases are settled privately by insurance companies or on the steps of the courts. Wherever the truth lies, it is clear that a fear of litigation is one of the challenges faced by the traditional cures in contemporary Ireland.

A few of my interviewees expressed concern about being sued by those they gave their cure to, especially if the cure had to be taken orally, like the man who most likely cured thousands of people of jaundice over many years with his herbal bottle. He had passed the cure to his daughter and she made it for a brief time, but stopped as she suspected that the land from which she took the herbs had become contaminated. Her father reflected, 'It's sad that the country has got so polluted that you can't even get a cure out of the ground anymore.' Another reason they called a halt to this old family cure was because of a worry regarding litigation. 'We got into a society ... that is very claim conscious ... There's no trust in people anymore,' he said. He believed that the herbal cures, particularly those that were taken as a beverage, were less likely to survive than the faith cures.

Another man I talked to, with a shingles cure, thought that many of the traditional cures were no longer being made as people were 'afraid of the legal aspect'. They were concerned that if someone had a negative reaction to their cure, they might be sued. And a man who had a faith cure for colic was reluctant to imply that he could cure the condition; 'I usually say ... I'll do my best for them, but I guarantee no cure ... You could be sued if you claimed to be making cures.' Nora Smyth found that a similar concern was expressed by some people with cures in Northern Ireland: 'I have even heard it said that many curers are afraid that they could leave themselves open to be sued by unsatisfied clients,' she wrote.

In the south-east there was a woman who made a skin cancer cure with plants. She too felt that a number of people could be reluctant to keep their cures going because they were fearful of being sued. She had this dilemma about her own cure, but continued to make it: 'You feel very bad if you can't help a person and you know that you should be able to.'

In 1986 I interviewed an old woman in rural Sligo who had a cure for piles. This was a herbal drink made from plants she gathered in the surrounding fields. She gave the cure to her daughter who lived close by and had a shop in the local town. When I went looking for this cure in 2006, I discovered that the old lady had died and her daughter no longer used it. This woman told me that she believed in cures, but that she had ceased making hers for two reasons; one person had complained that it made them sick and more importantly she was worried about being sued.

A farmer in Leitrim assured me that he had been cured of brucellosis by a woman in Laois many years previously. I managed to track down this elderly woman, who explained that it was a drink made from herbs she collected in her locality and that her mother had given her the cure. She had stopped making the cure because of 'rules and regulations' and she had no insurance cover for it. She said that she was afraid to keep producing her cure and had not passed it on. Also, I had heard of a well-respected herbal cure for skin cancer in north Mayo. This cure had been in the same family for generations and was passed from woman to man, to woman. I searched for the cure and found it in the possession of a female member of the family. Regretfully, she had decided to refrain from using it because of a fear of being sued; she was a solicitor!

There are other aspects of the law which have an influence on cures and traditional healing practice. The Donegal man who was the custodian of Gartan clay, used for protection and healing, gave it to people locally, nationally and internationally. In recent years he was aware that some people had been reluctant to bring it home with them to other countries, as they were nervous that this white, fine clay may be mistaken by airport customs as drugs.

I came across another matter of concern when I tried to visit a holy well in Kerry that had cures linked to it. I was disappointed to find that the entrance to this well was barred. I made enquiries nearby and was informed that a new landowner had blocked access to the holy well; a right that pilgrims had exercised for over 1,500 years. Hopefully this situation can be rectified swiftly, the right of way restored, and any indemnity issue the farmer had is addressed by the government.

## Plant Loss and Our Future

In the past in Ireland there was widespread use of plants to help and heal, as shown by the folklore gathered in the 1930s (The Schools' Collection). So-called weeds had and have a purpose; they exist for a reason and many of them can cure us. They are part of a complex, delicate and interdependent ecosystem. The following are a selection of well-known Irish plants and trees which have been used medicinally: hawthorn for hearts, herb-Robert for kidneys, plantain for burns, horsetail for bleeds, daisies for eyes, rushes for shingles, honeysuckle for jaundice, birch for eczema and ivy for inflammation. Niall Mac Coitir believes that 'plants are indispensable to our wellbeing. They feed us and heal (or harm) us, provide us with shelter and clothing, and nourish our souls with their beauty and tranquillity'.

A Leitrim farmer in his sixties had a herbal gallstones cure which his father had given to him. To make this traditional cure he ordered the herbs he needed from a supplier abroad. He thought that the old man who originally had the cure (in the 1950s) would have gathered the plants in the wild; 'long ago they grew here, if you knew what you were after'. Due to the mechanisation of Irish agriculture, he felt that 'herbs that grew along the roads ... they don't get a chance anymore ... they're gone'.

This area of concern (loss or contamination of plants used traditionally to heal) is part of a greater problem of habitat and biodiversity decline in Ireland and globally. David Bramwell, botanist and author, wrote in 1999 that, 'Mankind depends on plants to survive in the future, yet both locally and all over the world, we have a multitude of plants on the verge of disappearance as a consequence of human activity.'

Our planet is today facing two momentous, man-made, interconnected crises: climate change and biodiversity loss. In 2019 the Irish government acknowledged this reality and declared a Climate and Biodiversity Emergency. The enormous issues we have to deal with include: a dangerous increase in the earth's surface temperature, huge exploitation of our world's finite resources, wholesale destruction of nature, insatiable consumption, vast amounts of waste and endless pollution. The effects of climate change are upon us: melting icecaps, rising sea levels, greater frequency of severe floods, hurricanes, heatwaves, droughts, wildfires, harvest failures, hunger, population displacement and political instability. We are all affected, but more so the poorer countries which have less capability to deal with disasters.

The nations of the world came together to discuss these challenges and produced the Paris Agreement (2016). They agreed to pursue efforts to limit global warming to 1.5 degrees Celsius above pre-industrial levels.

The science is clear; we know what the problem is and how to address it. However, if we (in particular the richer, industrialised countries) do not start to radically change our way of living without delay, it will be too late. There will be catastrophic consequences for humanity and we will have destroyed our descendants' future.

A landmark UN (IPBES) global assessment report on biodiversity in 2019 made for grim reading. 'Biodiversity – the diversity within species, between species and of ecosystems – is declining faster than at any time in human history ... Nature across most of the globe has now been significantly altered by multiple human drivers ... around 1 million species already face extinction.' The study concluded that, 'Goals for conserving and sustainably using nature ... may only be achieved through transformative changes.' Following the publication of this report, ecologist Pádraic Fogarty from the Irish Wildlife Trust spoke to *The Irish Times* (7/5/19) about Ireland's biodiversity: 'Our seas have been emptied ... Nature has all but vanished from our hills, rivers and farmland due to pesticide use, wild fires, land drainage, pollution, plantations of conifers, reseeding and artificial fertilisation of soil and neglect of our ancient hedgerow network.'

I grew up on a farm, live in the heart of the countryside and feel very close to the land. We now need to consider the consequences of our actions upon it and look at how to reconnect with nature. We need to regain respect for the land and for all that is dependent upon it, including animals, birds, bees, trees and plants. Our use of the land must display this respect, working with nature, not against it.

We can also look to the past and reflect on the closeness our ancestors had to the natural world, how it sustained them, healed them and ensured their survival. Professor Proinsias Mac Cana has written that the Irish Celts were deeply connected to their land; 'Every river and lake and well, every plain and hill and mountain has its own name, and each name evokes its own explanatory legend.'

We need a new model for farming and land use in Ireland, one which keeps to the fore the huge problems our island and the world are facing. We could choose to move away from intensive agriculture and towards smaller-scale sustainable farming. Our farmers could produce much more food for the domestic market, a greater diversity of food and more plant-based food. There could be greater self-sufficiency on farms, a return to mixed farming, a focus on quality rather than quantity of food produced, and a determination to protect access to seed varieties and to contribute to global food security.

We must stop using herbicides, pesticides and synthetic fertilisers. Instead, we should prioritise the protection of soil fertility and our water sources, and animal welfare. Carbon storage has to be paramount; conserving the natural carbon stocks we have, rehabilitating the peatlands and planting native woodlands. Farmers could provide habitats that are pollinator friendly, encourage biodiversity and ecosystem regeneration.

Such an agricultural model would ensure that farming and rural communities can prosper and have a future. It would restore to us a landscape where wild plants can once again blossom and the traditional cures which come from them can be reclaimed. We could embrace as well the rewilding of much of our land and sea; this is the practice of protecting natural habitats and species from human exploitation, allowing them space and time to recover and flourish.

Collective action is required to address the climate change and biodiversity crises. Action has to take place at every level, individual, community, national and global. Sustainability must be kept at the centre of all public and private decision-making. Ensuring that our little country and our big planet move forward and thrive will necessitate creative thinking and vision, especially from our young people; it is theirs and their children's future which is at stake.

And we must always remember that each one of us is connected by the great web of Life, and that we share and depend on the natural world, fragile, beautiful and powerful. I leave the last word to Nemonte Nenquimo, Waorani tribal leader and land-rights campaigner, Ecuador. In 2019 she helped save her people's land (part of the Amazon rainforest, the richest source of herbal cures on earth) from oil drilling. The previous year she had sent out this message to all of us:

> as a woman, as a mother, as a water protector and a forest defender, I want you to join us in our fight to defend our way of life, our forests and our planet.

# Epilogue

🌿

THIS BOOK HAS TAKEN ME fifteen years to write. During that time the people I had met with cures and the practices associated with traditional healing in Ireland were never far from my thoughts. I see those I have interviewed as guardians of the cures, preserving and protecting them for future generations to benefit from. Cures may appear to be isolated and fragmented, with many individuals having a single one and usually no connection to others with cures. However, each person and each cure is part of a bigger picture, a healing tradition which goes back hundreds, probably thousands, of years. I see the cure as a separate entity to the person that is its current custodian, as having an independent existence, a life and history of its own.

It is amazing that the old cures have managed to survive despite the modernisation of Ireland and the immense changes that have taken place in our economy, society, culture and religious expression, including major medical advancements and technological developments. These cures work, not every time and not for everyone, but for many people, and this is the primary reason why they continue to exist. The cures live on because they are meeting a human need, more than a physical need, a psychological and a spiritual need too, and healing and good health incorporate these three elements. Modern medicine is not fulfilling all of people's healing needs, and this is reflected in the numerous forms of alternative medicines and therapies which are popular in Ireland today. The cures are part of this wider, more holistic approach to healing, and they have the strength of being deeply rooted in traditional culture.

I have documented one little-known aspect of Irish life at the commencement of the twenty-first century. I hope that my work will inspire others to make their own explorations into folk medicine, and the rich and fascinating folklore of Ireland. Those with cures should respect and protect them, and pass them on. Those of us who are not so fortunate should cherish their guardians and strive to keep the tradition alive.

> All the words that I utter,
> And all the words that I write,
> Must spread out their wings untiring,
> And never rest in their flight.

W.B. Yeats, 'Where My Books Go', 1892

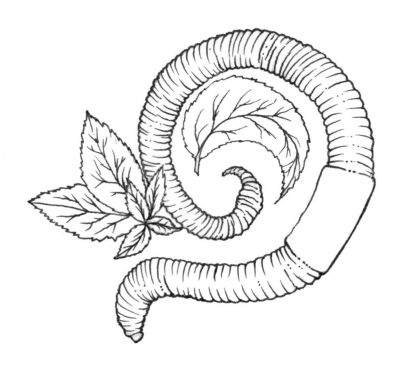

# Bibliography

Aalen, F.H.A., et al. (eds), *Atlas of the Irish Rural Landscape*, Cork University Press, Cork, 1997.

Achterberg, Jeanne, *Woman as Healer*, Rider Books, London, 1991.

Allen, David E. and Gabrielle Hatfield, *Medicinal Plants in Folk Tradition: An Ethnobotany of Britain and Ireland*, Timber Press, Portland, Oregon, 2004.

Attenborough, David, *A Life on Our Planet: My Witness Statement and a Vision for the Future*, Witness Books, London, 2020.

Barry, Margaret, et al. (eds), 'Lady Dudley's Scheme for the establishment of District Nurses in the poorest parts of Ireland', *Women's Studies Review*, Vol 5, National University of Ireland, Galway, 1997.

Bartram, Thomas, *Bartram's Encyclopedia of Herbal Medicine*, Robinson, London, 1998.

Beach, Russell P. (ed.), *AA Touring Guide to Ireland*, The Automobile Association, Hampshire, England, 1976.

Beckett, J.C., *The Making of Modern Ireland 1603–1923*, Faber and Faber, London, 1969.

Blake, Liam (photography), Fintan O'Toole (introduction), *Shrines*, Real Ireland Design, Wicklow, 2001.

Blake, R. Marlay, 'Folk Lore: With some account of the Ancient Gaelic Leeches and the state of the Art of Medicine in Ancient Erin', *Journal of the County Louth Archaeological Society*, Vol 4, No 3, Dundalk, December 1918.

Bord, Janet and Colin, *Sacred Waters: Holy Wells and Water Lore in Britain and Ireland*, Granada, London, 1985.

— *The Secret Country*, Granada, London, 1978.

Bourke, Angela, *The Burning of Bridget Cleary: A True Story*, Pimlico, London, 1999.

Branigan, Gary, *Ancient and Holy Wells of Dublin*, The History Press, Dublin, 2012.

Breen, Richard, 'The Ritual Expression of Inter-Household Relationships in Ireland', *Cambridge Anthropology*, Vol 6, England, 1980.

Buckley, Anthony D., 'Unofficial Healing in Ulster', *Ulster Folklife*, Vol 26, Ulster Folk and Transport Museum, Co. Down, 1980.

Carr, Peter, *The Night of the Big Wind*, The White Row Press, Belfast, 1993.

Chadwick, Nora, *The Celts*, Penguin Books, Middlesex, England, 1970.

Claffey, Patrick (text), Bereska Tomasz and Szustek Tomasz (photography), *Atlantic Tabor: The Pilgrims of Croagh Patrick*, The Liffey Press, Dublin, 2016.

Condren, Mary, *The Serpent and the Goddess: Women, Religion and Power in Celtic Ireland*, New Island Books, Dublin, second edition, 2002.

Conlon-McKenna, Marita, *Under the Hawthorn Tree*, The O'Brien Press, Dublin, 1990.

Corrigan, Desmond, 'The scientific basis of folk medicine: The Irish dimension', *Plant Lore Studies*, No 18, Folklore Society of London University, 1984.

Creedon, John, *An Irish Folklore Treasury: A Selection of Old Stories, Ways and Wisdom from the Schools' Collection*, Gill Books, Dublin, 2022.

Cronin, Phil, *Traditional Cures and Gifted People*, Mayo, 2002.

Culpeper, Nicholas, *Culpeper's Complete Herbal*, Foulsham and Co., London, 1964.

Curley, Helen (ed.), *Local Ireland Almanac and Yearbook of Facts 2000*, Local Ireland, Dublin, 1999.

Danaher, Kevin, 'Ancient Healers', *Biatas: The Tillage Farmer*, Carlow, September 1963.

— 'The Herb Doctors', *Biatas*, June 1966.

— 'The Healing Art', *Biatas*, October 1966.

— *Irish Customs and Beliefs*, Mercier Press, Cork, 2004.

Day, Robert, 'Folk-lore', *The Journal of the Royal Historical and Archaeological Association of Ireland*, Vol 8, Dublin, 1888.

Delaney, Frank, *The Celts*, Grafton, London, 1989.

Dent, J. Geoffrey, 'The Irish reputation for healing in Northern England', *Ulster Folklife*, Vol 14, Ulster Folk and Transport Museum, Co. Down, 1968.

De Vries, Jan, *Traditional Home and Herbal Remedies*, Mainstream, Edinburgh, 1986.

Doherty, Michael L., 'The folklore of cattle diseases: A veterinary perspective', *Béaloideas: Journal of the Folklore of Ireland Society*, Vol 69, Dublin, 2001.

Dowd, Marion, *The Archaeology of Caves in Ireland*, Oxbow Books, Oxford, 2015.

Doyle, Bill (photography), Muiris Mac Conghail (text), *Island Funeral*, Veritas, Dublin, 2000.

Ennybegs Irish Countrywomen's Association, *A Collection of Cures, Remedies and Miscellany*, self-published, Longford, 2003.

Evans, E. Estyn, *Irish Folk Ways*, Routledge and Kegan Paul, London, 1957.

Evans Wentz, W.Y., *The Fairy-Faith in Celtic Countries*, Colin Smythe, Buckinghamshire, England, 1977.

Flanagan, Deirdre and Laurence, *Irish Place Names*, Gill & Macmillan, Dublin, 2002.

Fleetwood, John, *History of Medicine in Ireland*, Browne and Nolan, Dublin, 1951.

Flower, Robin, *The Irish Tradition*, Clarendon Press, Oxford, 1947.

Flynn, Laurence, 'St Patrick's Purgatory: Lough Derg, County Donegal', *The Irish Heritage Series*, 54, Eason and Sons, Dublin, 1987.

Fogarty, Pádraic, *Whittled Away: Ireland's Vanishing Nature*, The Collins Press, Cork, 2017.

Friel, Brian, *Dancing at Lughnasa*, Farrar, Straus and Giroux, New York, 1998.

Gallagher, Emer, et al., *Tóchar Phádraig: A Pilgrim's Progress, Ballintubber to Croagh Patrick*, Ballintubber Abbey Publication, Mayo, 1989.

Gallagher, Fióna, *The Streets of Sligo: Urban Evolution Over the Course of Seven Centuries*, Fióna Gallagher, Burton Street, self-published, Sligo, 2008.

Gallagher, Michael, *Remedies and Cures of Bygone Era*, self-published, Donegal, 2012.

Gantz, Jeffrey (trans.), *Early Irish Myths and Sagas*, Penguin Books, London, 1981.

Gillespie, Christy, *St Colm Cille, Gartan to Iona: A Life's Journey*, self-published, Donegal, 1997.

Glassie, Henry, *Passing the Time: Folklore and History of an Ulster Community*, O'Brien Press, Dublin, 1982.

Graves, Robert, *The White Goddess: A Historical Grammar of Poetic Myth*, Farrar, Straus and Giroux, New York, 2013.

Gregory, Lady, *Gods and Fighting Men*, Colin Smythe, Buckinghamshire, England, 1976.

— *Visions and Beliefs in the West of Ireland*, Colin Smythe, Buckinghamshire, England, 1976.

Grieve, Mrs M., *A Modern Herbal*, Penguin Books, Middlesex, England, 1980.

Harbison, Peter, *Pilgrimage in Ireland: The Monuments and the People*, Barrie and Jenkins, London, 1991.

Healy, Elizabeth, *In Search of Ireland's Holy Wells*, Wolfhound Press, Dublin, 2001.

Heaney, Marie, *Over Nine Waves: A Book of Irish Legends*, Faber and Faber, London, 1995.

Heraughty, Patrick, *Inishmurray: Ancient monastic island*, O'Brien Press, Dublin, 1982.

— Interview with Cecily Gilligan, Sligo, 1 January 1986.

Herity, Michael, *Gleanncholmcille: A guide to 5,000 years of history in stone*, Na Clocha Breaca, Dublin, 1998.

— *Rathcroghan and Carnfree*, Na Clocha Breaca, Dublin, 1991.

Hickie, David (text), Mike O' Toole (photography), Austin Carey (illustrations), *Native Trees and Forests of Ireland*, Gill & Macmillan, Dublin, 2002.

Hoffmann, David, *Welsh Herbal Medicine*, Abercastle Publications, Ceredigion, Wales, 2000.

Hunt, Harriet J.H., 'A folk-cure from Donegal', *Béaloideas: Journal of the Folklore of Ireland Society*, Vol 3, Dublin, 1932.

Hurston, Zora Neale, *The Sanctified Church*, Turtle Island, Berkeley, California, 1981.

Hyde, Douglas, *Beside the Fire: A Collection of Irish Gaelic Folk Stories*, Forgotten Books, London, 2007.

IPBES (Intergovernmental Science-Policy Platform on Biodiversity and Ecosystem Services), *The Global Assessment Report on Biodiversity and Ecosystem Services*, Bonn, Germany, 2019.

Jackson, Kenneth H., *A Celtic Miscellany*, Penguin Books, Middlesex, England, 1971.

Jaén, José, *Handbook of Canary Folk Medicine: The Secrets of Our Old Herbalists*, Centro de la Cultura Popular Canaria, Gran Canaria, 1999.

Jarvis, D.C., *Folk Medicine*, Crest Books, New York, 1962.

Jenkins, Richard P., 'Witches and Fairies: Supernatural Aggression and Deviance among the Irish Peasantry', *Ulster Folklife*, Vol 23, Ulster Folk and Transport Museum, Co. Down, 1977.

Jones, Anne E., 'Folk Medicine in Living Memory in Wales', *Folk Life: Journal of Ethnological Studies*, Vol 18, Swansea, Wales, 1980.

Kaptchuk, Ted, and Michael Croucher, *The Healing Arts: A Journey Through the Faces of Medicine*, British Broadcasting Corporation, London, 1986.

Kavanagh, Peter, *Irish Mythology: A Dictionary*, Goldsmith Press, Kildare, 1988.

Kennedy L., et al., *Mapping the Great Irish Famine: A Survey of the Famine Decades*, Four Courts Press, Dublin, 1999.

Kilgannon, Tadhg, *Sligo and its Surroundings*, Kilgannon and Sons, Sligo, 1926.

Kindred, Glennie, *Sacred Celebrations: A Sourcebook*, Gothic Image, Glastonbury, 2007.

Kingston, Rosari, 'Folk Medicine and Its Second Life', *Journal of Irish Studies*, University College Cork, 31 October 2017.

— 'A Tale of Two Bone-setters', *Béascna: Journal of Folklore and Ethnology*, Vol 8, University College Cork, 2013.

Kinsella, Thomas (trans.), Louis Le Brocquy (drawings), *The Táin*, Oxford University Press, London and The Dolmen Press, Dublin, 1970.

Kroll, Una, *In Touch with Healing*, BBC Books, London, 1991.

Lenihan, Edmund, *In Search of Biddy Early*, Mercier Press, Cork, 1987.

Lewton-Brain, James, 'Witches and Gender', *UCG Women's Studies Centre Review*, Vol 3, University College Galway, 1995.

Logan, Patrick, *Irish Country Cures*, Appletree Press, Belfast, 1981.

— *The Holy Wells of Ireland*, Colin Smythe, Buckinghamshire, England, 1980

— *The Old Gods: The Facts about Irish Fairies*, Appletree Press, Belfast, 1981.

— 'Folk medicine of the Cavan–Leitrim area', *Ulster Folklife*, Vol 9, 1963 and Vol 11, 1965.

Loughrey, Patrick (ed.), *The People of Ireland*, Appletree Press, Belfast, 1988.

Mabey, Richard, *Food for Free*, Collins, London, 1972.

— *Nature Cure*, Pimlico, London, 2006.

Mac Cabe, Niamh, 'Tor Mór's Trinity Knot', *Sligo Field Club Journal*, Vol 4, Sligo, 2018.

Mac Cana, Proinsias, *Celtic Mythology*, Hamlyn, London, 1970.

Mac Coitir, Niall, *Irish Trees: Myths, Legends and Folklore*, The Collins Press, Cork, 2003.

— *Irish Wild Plants: Myths, Legends and Folklore*, The Collins Press, Cork, 2006.

MacFarlane, Anne, 'The changing role of women as health workers in Ireland', *Women's Studies Review*, Vol 5, National University of Ireland, Galway, 1997.

Macfarlane, Robert (text), Jackie Morris (illustrations), *The Lost Words: A Spell Book*, Hamish Hamilton, London, 2017.

MacLochlainn, Cóilín, *Tory Island: A Visitor's Guide*, Comharchumann Thoraí Teo, Donegal, 2003.

MacManus, Seumas, *The Story of the Irish Race*, Wings Books, New Jersey, USA, 1990.

MacNeill, Máire, *The Festival of Lughnasa: A Study of the Survival of the Celtic Festival of the Beginning of Harvest*, Comhairle Bhéaloideas Éireann, University College Dublin, 2008.

Mahon, Bríd, *While Green Grass Grows: Memoirs of a Folklorist*, Mercier Press, Cork, 1998.

Maloney, Beatrice, 'Traditional Herbal Cures in County Cavan: Part 1', *Ulster Folklife*, Vol 18, Ulster Folk and Transport Museum, Co. Down, 1972.

Mc Glynn, Martina (presenter), Daly Garret (producer), Liam O'Brien (production supervisor), 'A Light from the Grave', *Documentary on One*, RTÉ Radio 1, Dublin, first broadcast 9 July 2006.

McGuire, Peter, 'Magical mystery cures', *The Irish Times*, 26 October 2013.

Meehan, Pádraig, *Listoghil: A Seasonal Alignment? Interpreting Carrowmore at the Heart of Neolithic Sligo*, Gungho Publications, Leitrim, 2013.

Mitchell, Frank and Michael Ryan, *Reading the Irish Landscape*, Town House, Dublin, 1998.

Moloney, Michael F., *Irish Ethno-Botany and the Evolution of Medicine in Ireland*, Gill and Son, Dublin, 1919.

Moore, Ronnie, *A General Practice, A Country Practice: The Cure, the Charm and Informal Healing in Northern Ireland*, Folk Healing and Health Care Practices in Britain and Ireland, Berghahn Books, Oxford, 2010.

Moore, Sam (ed.), *Sligo, Land of the Heart's Desire: Driving Tours and Short Walks*, Highwood Community Resource Centre, Sligo, 1999.

Morris, Henry, 'Cassidy's Rag: The Growth of a Superstition', *Journal of the County Louth Archaeological Society*, Vol 3, Dundalk, 1914.

Muir, Tom, *The Mermaid Bride and Other Orkney Folk Tales*, Kirkwall Press, Orkney, 1998.

Murphy, Dervla, *Tibetan Foothold*, Eland Publishing, London, 2011.

National Folklore Collection, *The Schools' Collection*, 1937–39, Vol 664, p. 85, Vol 1096, p. 175, Vol 230, p. 35, Vol 789, p. 271, University College Dublin, www.dúchas.ie, accessed 13 February 2021.

Nenquimo, Nemonte, 'The Ceibo Alliance: Protecting Indigenous Land in the Amazon Rainforest from Big Oil', National Bioneers Conference, California, USA, 20 October 2018.

Ní Fhloinn, Bairbre, 'From medieval text to mobile: Folk medicine in Irish tradition', lecture, Royal Irish Academy, Dublin, 24 August 2016.

Nolan, Peter W., 'Folk Medicine in Rural Ireland', *Folk Life*, Vol 27, Swansea, Wales, 1989.

Oakley, Ann, 'Wisewoman and Medicine Man: Changes in the Management of Childbirth', in *The Rights and Wrongs of Women*, Penguin Books, Middlesex, England, 1976.

O'Brien, Edna, *Mother Ireland*, Penguin Books, Middlesex, England, 1978.

Ó Crualaoich, Gearóid, *The Book of The Cailleach: Stories of the Wise-Woman Healer*, Cork University Press, Cork, 2003.

O'Dowd, Anne, *Straw, Hay and Rushes in Irish Folk Tradition*, Irish Academic Press, Dublin, 2015.

O'Farrell, Padraic, *Irish Folk Cures*, and *Irish Customs*, Gill & Macmillan, Dublin, 2004.

Ó Héalaí, Pádraig, 'Pregnancy and Childbirth in Blasket Island Tradition', *Women's Studies Review*, Vol 5, National University of Ireland, Galway, 1997.

Ó hÓgáin, Dáithí, *The Lore of Ireland: An Encyclopaedia of Myth, Legend and Romance*, The Collins Press, Cork, 2006.

— *The Sacred Isle: Belief and Religion in Pre-Christian Ireland*, The Boydell Press, Suffolk and The Collins Press, Cork, 1999.

O'Regan, Paula, *Healing Herbs in Ireland*, Primrose Press, Dublin, 1997.

Ó Súilleabháin, Seán, *A Handbook of Irish Folklore*, Singing Tree Press, Detroit, 1970.

O'Toole, Edward, 'A Miscellany of North Carlow Folklore', *Béaloideas: Journal of the Folklore of Ireland Society*, Vol 1, Dublin, 1928.

Owen, Alex, *The Darkened Room: Women, Power and Spiritualism in Late Victorian England*, Virago Press, London, 1989.

Podlech, Dieter, *Herbs and Healing Plants of Britain and Europe*, Harper Collins, London, 2010.

Purdon, Henry S., 'Notes on Old Native Remedies', *The Dublin Journal of Medical Science*, Vol C, Dublin, 1895.

— 'Note on an old "Surgical" Remedy', *Ulster Journal of Archaeology*, Vol 2, Queen's University Belfast, 1896.

Quinn, Bob, *The Atlantean Irish: Ireland's Oriental and Maritime Heritage*, The Lilliput Press, Dublin, 2005.

Rackard, Anna and Liam O'Callaghan, *Fish, Stone, Water: Holy Wells of Ireland*, Atrium, Cork, 2001.

Reader, Ian, *Making Pilgrimages: Meaning and Practice in Shikoku*, University of Hawaii Press, Honolulu, 2005.

Roberts, Jack, *The Sheela-na-gigs of Ireland: An Illustrated Map and Guide*, Bandia Publishing, Galway, 2009.

Ross, Gyasi, 'History, Biology and Purpose – What it means to be a member of a Native community' (Christine Quintasket quote), Community Wellness Conference, Tulalip, Washington, USA, Tulalip News, 20 May 2015.

Ryan, Meda, *Biddy Early: The Wise Woman of Clare*, Mercier Press, Cork, 1978.

Scallan, Christine, *Irish Herbal Cures*, Newleaf, Dublin, 1994.

Schmitz, Nancy, 'An Irish Wise Woman: Fact and legend', *Journal of the Folklore Institute*, Vol 14, Indiana University Press, USA, 1977.

Severin, Tim, *The Brendan Voyage*, Arrow Books, London, 1979.

Skidmore-Roth, Linda, *Mosby's Handbook of Herbs and Natural Supplements*, Elsevier, St Louis, USA, fourth edition, 2009.

Slavin, Michael, *The Book of Tara*, Wolfhound Press, Dublin, 2002.

Smyth, Nora, *Going for the Cure: Traditional Cures in Co. Armagh*, self-published, Armagh, 2002.

Speirs, Derek, *Pavee Pictures*, Dublin Travellers Education and Development Group, Dublin, 1991.

Szövérffy, Joseph, 'The Well of the Holy Women: Some St. Columba traditions in the West of Ireland', *Journal of American Folklore*, Vol 68, University of Illinois Press, USA, 1955.

Therman, Dorothy Harrison, *Stories from Tory Island*, Country House, Dublin, 1989.

Thunberg, Greta, *No One is Too Small to Make a Difference*, Penguin Books, London, 2019.

Tucker, Vincent, 'From Biomedicine to Holistic Health: Towards a New Health Model', *The Sociology of Health and Illness in Ireland*, University College Dublin Press, Dublin, 1997.

UCD Library Cultural Heritage Collections, 'Sphagnum Moss to the rescue', University College Dublin, 28 June 2018.

Unknown author, *Dictionary of the Celts*, Geddes and Grosset, Scotland, 1999.

Waddell, John, *The Prehistoric Archaeology of Ireland*, Wordwell, Bray, Wicklow, 2000.

Wilde, Lady, *Ancient Legends, Mystic Charms, and Superstitions of Ireland*, Ward and Downey, London, 1888.

Wilson, T.G., 'Some Irish folklore remedies for diseases of the ear, nose and throat', *Irish Journal of Medical Science*, Vol 18, Dublin, 1943.

Woodham-Smith, Cecil, *The Great Hunger, Ireland 1845–1849*, Penguin Books, London, 1991.

World Health Organization, *WHO Traditional Medicine Strategy 2014–2023*, www.who. int, accessed 12 May 2023.

Yeats, W.B. (ed.), *Fairy and Folk Tales of Ireland*, Colin Smythe, Buckinghamshire, England, 1995.

— *Selected Poetry*, Macmillan, London, 1970.

Youngson, Robert, *The Royal Society of Medicine Health Encyclopedia*, Bloomsbury, London, 2000.

# Index

# About the Author

**C**ECILY GILLIGAN GREW UP AND lives in rural County Sligo. She is a primary school teacher and has a degree in Social Science and a Masters in Women's Studies from University College Cork. She has been interested in folklore since childhood, when much of her knowledge was acquired from within her community, and in particular from her grandmother. Cecily is a world traveller, a sailor and a hillwalker. She has a love of Irish culture and history, and the Irish language. She is a campaigner for the protection of human rights and the environment, locally and globally.

# Acknowledgements

THANK YOU TO ALL THOSE with cures who generously shared their thoughts and experiences with me. The many more who helped me during my research and travels around Ireland. My late husband Andy for his love and support, and for inspiring me to start this book many moons ago. My late mother Angela for her love and positivity. The late Vincent Tucker, my mentor and outstanding lecturer at University College Cork.

Thanks to my friends for their love, advice and practical help, in particular Niamh, Mary Mc, Paula, Rosemarie, Luke and Chris. My nieces and nephews, always remembering little Eoin, and Tom, a gentleman. My dear neighbours no longer with us, Paddy, Mary Kate and Bridgie. My little dog Ruby who accompanied me on so many adventures. Nora, Johnny and Waters Cottage. The Merrion Press team – Conor, Patrick, Heidi, Wendy, Maeve and Conor Holbrook, and Karen Vaughan for her wonderful illustrations. Bairbre Ní Fhloinn, Associate Professor of the School of Irish, Celtic Studies and Folklore, University College Dublin, for her support for my research. Auri and the good people of La Restinga, El Hierro. Fiona, PJ, Rietje and the beautiful Burren.

*Go raibh míle maith agaibh*